HEALING
SECRETS
OF THE
SEASONS

other books by judith benn hurley

Savoring the Day

The Good Herb

Garden-Fresh Cooking

Healthy Microwave Cooking

The Healing Foods
(Patti Hausman, coauthor)

The Healthy Gourmet
(Patti Hausman, coauthor)

The Surgeon General's Report on Nutrition and Health
(Patti Hausman, coauthor)

HEALING SECRETS OF THE SEASONS

*recipes and remedies that
soothe, de-stress, and energize
throughout the year*

JUDITH BENN HURLEY

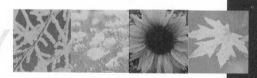

WILLIAM MORROW AND COMPANY, INC. | NEW YORK

It is the policy of William Morrow and Company, Inc., and its
imprints and affiliates, recognizing the importance of preserving
what has been written, to print the books we publish on acid-
free paper, and we exert our best efforts to that end.

Library of Congress Cataloging-in-Publication Data

Hurley, Judith Benn.
    Healing secrets of the seasons : recipes and remedies that
    soothe, de-stress, and energize throughout the year / Judith
    Benn Hurley.
        p.   cm.
    Includes index.
    ISBN 0-688-15435-2
    1. Nutrition—Popular works.   2. Food habits—Popular
works.   3. Health—Popular works.   4. Self-care, Health—
Popular works.   I. Title.
RA784.H865   1998
613.2—dc21   98-3896
                    CIP

Printed in the United States of America

First Edition

1   2   3   4   5   6   7   8   9   10

BOOK DESIGN BY DEBBIE GLASSERMAN

www.williammorrow.com

for patrick

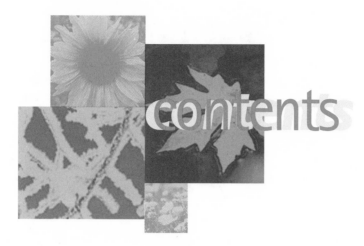

contents

acknowledgments

It was an honor for me to work with Toni Sciarra, Katharine Cluverius, Ann Cahn, Debbie Glasserman, and all the hardworking people at William Morrow; Susan Chaires; Dr. Bob and the Buddha Girls; and The Chinaman.

For research and testing, I thank Stan Benn, Jo Ann Brader, Gail Concannon, Linda Cucher, Cindy Kettell, Nancy Langsdale, Judy Lieberman, Lori Settimi, Liz Scarlett, Mary Kay Scarlett, Susan Stanton, Jan Wilcox, and Nancy Zelko.

before
you begin
this book

the secret to living well is adopting a harmonious compromise with nature. For a simple example, when outside temperatures plummet, we slip on extra clothes to maintain normal body heat and avoid illness. Similarly, in hot weather we shed heavy clothing, and eat lighter, high-water-content foods to keep ourselves cool, comfortable, and healthy. Harmonious compromise—there is great power in this very simple concept, and it is the essence of *Healing Secrets of the Seasons*.

But this is not a new notion.

Thousands of years ago, on the banks of the Tigris and Nile rivers, women began making notes about how their bodies changed according to the seasons. On wooden sticks that represented a year, they recorded twelve lunar cycles that concurred with their own twenty-eight-day cycles. Near appropriate moons they carved symbols for when the earth was cold and still; when the earth came to life with sprouts and blossoms; when animals migrated; when various plants were harvested; and how a woman's body and mind changed along with the seasons. The women showed their sticks to tribal leaders, usually men, who realized that the potent information the sticks provided could, in a sense, foretell the future, thus helping to create a good and healthy life. Egyptian priests called the sticks "Fingers of the Sun," while others called them "magic wands."

Egyptians then began carving their seasonal information on stone slabs, while Norse, Dane, and Celtic carvers preferred wood made into blocks, called "clogs." By the twelfth century, seasonal information was chronicled on parchment and included holidays, navigational data, proverbs, agricultural information, health tips, astrology, and recipes. These were the first publications of many societies, and were the earliest versions of what we now refer to as calendars and almanacs.

Some early societies probed even deeper into the seasonal impact on human health. The Greek physician Hippocrates instructed his medical students to "consider the seasons of the year and what effect each of them produces" when diagnosing illness. Also seasonally oriented, early Chinese physicians developed the Five Elements Theory, part of which reports how our bodies and minds change at different seasons, noting, for instance, that winter may produce feelings of depression and summer may bring joy.

Of the same thread are modern scientists who recognize a condition called "seasonal affective disorder" (SAD) that can occur as winter approaches. As daylight hours diminish, some people become depressed and lethargic. But knowing in advance that this and other seasonal states may occur can help us prepare to stay healthy. What's more, by observing seasonal changes we keep in touch with the natural world around us, grounding and balancing ourselves as we whirl toward the coming century.

using this book

With *Healing Secrets of the Seasons* I have in a sense carved my own calendar stick, using food, herbs, and healing arts to stay balanced and healthy in each of the four seasons, and during the transitions between them.

Healing Secrets of the Seasons contains four large chapters, one for each season of the year. Each chapter includes activities that are best done during that season; interesting dates for each month in the season; a First Aid Kit offering ideas for remedies and activities to promote seasonal well-being; beverage recipes to help prevent and cure seasonal ills; best foods to eat during the season, including quick cooking tips, recipes, and seasonal menu suggestions.

To incorporate this information into your daily life, simply open *Healing Secrets of the Seasons* to the current season. Let's say it's autumn. You'll discover that gathering, building, and storing are the activities that define the season, and you'll glean advice on the foods, herbs, and activities that will help strengthen you and prevent such autumn maladies as colds, coughs, and flu.

Healing Secrets of the Seasons also offers four smaller "Gateway" chapters between the large seasonal ones, featuring tips on how to stay healthy during the transition of the seasons. Navajo, Chinese, and other healers believe that these "gateways" of change can become times of stress, making people more susceptible to sickness. Anyone who has ever caught an early fall cold might agree! So if it is autumn, in addition to consulting the Autumn chapter, you would also refer to the Gateway chapters from Summer to Autumn and from Autumn to Winter.

What fascinated me most while doing research for *Healing Secrets of the Seasons* was the common thread in the wisdom offered to me by dozens of healers throughout the world—Chinese, Caribbean, Ayurvedic, Navajo, Cherokee, Lenape, English, Hawaiian, Irish, Welsh, Egyptian, Japanese, Brazilian, Italian, French, Indonesian, Filipino, and African: For maximum well-being, heed the seasons.

Healing Secrets of the Seasons gives you the knowledge to apply that advice each day. In addition, the book is flavored with another philosophy I learned from these many wise people: What you get out of a particular season has a lot to do with what you put into it. For instance, instead of speculating what summer has to offer you, explore what *you* can bring to summer. Positivism, for example, would be a useful attitude to bring to any season, enhancing your outlook and ultimately your health and well-being. I hope you will experiment with these theories. Here's how.

Tug at one thing in nature,
and discover it is connected to
an entire universe.

JOHN MUIR

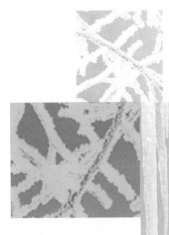

winter:
the season
of rest

november, december, january

BEST TIME OF YEAR FOR:

❋ *Rest, repose, and relaxation*

❋ *Digging deep into yourself*

❋ *Dreaming*

as the sun disappeared behind the pyramids one December evening, I arrived at a party in Cairo, Egypt, wearing a light evening dress and a silk shawl tossed carelessly over one shoulder.

"You must be *freezing*!" my hostess squealed.

"Oh, I'm *fine*, it's a gorgeous seventy-five degrees," I replied, confused.

"But it's *winter*!" she reminded, as if I didn't know the meaning of the word.

As a child, winter to me meant icy, windy days, with mounds of snow. But I have since known winter in England where the weather was merely balmy, and where because of the northern latitude, the sun set at three in the afternoon. A Malaysian winter, I discovered, means one hundred-degree heat with daily tropical storms.

No matter where you winter, however, the trademark of the season is shorter days. That means fewer daylight hours, and since natural light helps us feel balanced and energized, many people experience a corresponding tendency toward winter irritability and depression. This is especially true when we overcommit and expect too much of ourselves—if, say, excessive activity is crammed into this shorter span of daytime. The solution is to be in rhythm with the winter season by adopting a calmly active pace.

THE MONTH OF NOVEMBER Our eleventh month was named for the number nine, because it was the ninth month in the old Roman calendar. In literature, to be "Novemberish" is to be misty and mysterious.

WINTER: THE SEASON OF REST

3

INTERESTING DATES IN NOVEMBER

November 11—Feast of Bacchus in ancient Rome where people dined on winter grains and vegetables, and paid off their debts with money made from harvests. *November 13—Feast of Jupiter* in ancient Rome, when people ate together and toasted to seal winter commitments. *November 21* (approximate)—The sun enters the zodiac sign of Sagittarius, the Archer, ruled by the planet Jupiter, symbolizing friendly and ambitious attitudes.

THE MONTH OF DECEMBER The twelfth month in our calendar is from the Latin *decem*, meaning "ten," because December was the tenth month in the old Roman year. Throughout the world December is the month for winter festivities and joy. Owls and evergreens are literary symbols of December.

One example of extreme winter slow-down is the bear, who hibernates during this dimly lit season. But observe your local fauna and discover that all animals instinctively slow down for winter. Street squirrels are barely visible, because most of the time they're at rest in cozy tree nests. Racehorses, including those who reside in warm Miami, Florida, are sometimes slower in winter. Even house pets—cats and dogs—are less active than in brighter seasons.

Ancient African and bedouin tribes knew this rhythm and began their calendar years in winter, as we do now, because it provided a time for leisure and celebrations after the rigorous harvest season. Early Japanese societies called winter the "white season," or "silver world," which they associated with restfulness and Zen meditation. In classic Chinese art and literature the symbol for winter is the tortoise, for its steady yet unhurried pace. And in North America some Indian tribes made a "winter count" during this less active season, which was a quietly created pictorial or written reflection of the year's events. One modern version of slowing down might be a more internal activity such as keeping a journal, instead of taking tennis lessons.

This does not mean that you should cease physical activity during winter. Experts advise staying active with such pursuits as walking, skiing, yoga, or tai chi, which help increase circulation, keeping you warm and energized. In addition, winter exercise will help prevent unwanted weight gain during this more restful and inward-directed time. You may also wish to use some of the soothing tips, teas, and foods below, to create a warming balance for yourself during this season of repose.

first aid kit for winter

The assortment of items and ideas that follow can help you create a peaceful and interesting season. They are easy to adopt into your own rhythm, and you may have already embraced one or two on your own.

Warm Your Heart—Keep cut flowers and green plants around your home and office. Flowers are beautiful, uplifting to your mood, and they create a cheerful atmosphere. Green plants soothe the eye and help freshen the air you breathe. Try a spider plant or pothos (it looks like a philodendron but the leaves are marbled with creamy white), which are easy to grow in most environments.

Warm Your Mind—Stock up on thought-provoking reading material for long winter nights. Try Ralph Waldo Emerson's *Essays* or the *Great Dialogues of Plato*. Browse in your local library or bookstore for subjects that you've never had a chance to explore. You may also wish to join a book club that meets regularly to discuss a specific title. If there's no club in your area, start one according to your own reading interests—mysteries, or perhaps romances.

Warm Your Body—To soothe winter aches and pains, keep a supply of bath oils, bath salts, and aromatic soaps for soaking in the tub. Natural essences of pine, eucalyptus, rosemary, thyme, or birch will temporarily relieve the pain from sore muscles and joints, and many products are available in all price ranges. Also readily available are potions to soothe winter stresses, containing lavender, chamomile, orange blossom, sandalwood, or marjoram, available at pharmacies, department stores, natural food stores, herb shops, and many supermarkets. To make your own blend, run a warm bath and swirl in a cup of Epsom salts, available at pharmacies. Then add about a teaspoon of canola oil to help soften your skin. Before you step in to soak, add about five drops of essential oil of lavender (or essence of your choice). Soak for about twenty minutes, then lightly towel dry, leaving your skin moist. Rub a soothing, aromatic skin oil or lotion onto your damp skin (for better absorption), then bundle up and relax for the evening. Note that if your skin is itchy from being overly dry, skip the salt bath and take a comforting oat bath instead. Colloidal oatmeal or oats that dissolve in bathwater are available at most pharmacies. Add five drops of essential oil of lavender for a supremely soothing treatment.

Warm the World—Forget about your own problems and do something for someone else. If you have an extra coat, give it to someone

December 22 (approximate)—The sun enters the zodiac sign of Capricorn, the Goat, symbolizing a focused and organized mind. This day also marks the winter solstice, or the longest night of the year. *Geminid Meteor Shower* (date floats)—Check your local paper for the exact night of this celestial event, when lovely silver streaks decorate the sky every ten to thirty seconds. *December 31—Demon-Ousting Day* in Japan, when incense sticks are burned to rid the house of demons and freshen up for the new calendar year.

THE MONTH OF JANUARY

Our first calendar month is named for Janus, Roman god of gates and doors, openings, and all beginnings. This is a splendid month in which to plan a change.

who needs it. Many dry cleaners collect coats for the needy, so check with yours. Sort out toys that aren't being used and give them to one of the many agencies that distribute to children who have none. If you do just one thing this season, such as giving time, money, or food to those who need it more than you, it may put your own winter worries into perspective.

INTERESTING DATES IN JANUARY

January 1—Feast of Janus in ancient Rome, where candles were lit to inspire good luck to new ventures begun this year. *January 6—Twelfth Night*, marking the last night of the Yule season. You may wish to adopt the French custom and bake a cake with a bean hidden inside. She or he whose piece of cake holds the bean is said to have a lucky year ahead.

soothing winter beverages

The natural rhythm of the seasons may have already led you to choose such soothing, warming beverages as spiced orange tea or ginger tea. Another easy winter remedy to increase circulation, clear a stuffy head, and take a chill off the body is to swirl your favorite coffee or black tea with a fragrant vanilla bean. Or, as the days become shorter and temperatures drop, try these tasty and comforting brews.

after-holiday digestive tonic

To settle your stomach after overindulging in the season's delicacies, drink this delicious and refreshing potion. The secret ingredient is herbal bitters, in which the main component, gentian root, helps to stimulate digestion and dispel intestinal gas.

½ cup chilled orange juice
½ cup chilled seltzer water

1 to 2 teaspoons bitters (such as angostura bitters, available at supermarkets)

If the weather is damp: Use the full 2 teaspoons of bitters.

If the weather is dry: Add a slice of lemon before drinking.

Combine all of the ingredients in a glass and drink after a meal.

MAKES 1 SERVING; 60 CALORIES; NO ADDED FAT.

warming ginger nectar

If the weather is damp: Add a 2-inch cinnamon stick before simmering, then discard.

If the weather is dry: Add a teaspoon lemon juice to each serving before drinking.

Prepare this tonic when you feel withered and fatigued. The gingerroot will help to energize you gently, and the licorice root promotes hydration of the skin and intestines. If you have high blood pressure, omit the licorice, as it may aggravate the condition.

10 slices fresh gingerroot
¼ cup Chinese dried jujube fruits
   or raisins

3 slices dried Chinese licorice root
6 cups water

In a medium saucepan, combine all of the ingredients and bring to a boil. Reduce the heat to medium-low, cover loosely, and simmer for about 20 minutes. Discard the roots and fruit and sip warm. You can make this beverage ahead and take it to work in a Thermos to refresh your day.

MAKES 4 SERVINGS; 30 CALORIES PER SERVING; NO ADDED FAT.

carrot-peppermint stomach soother

If the weather is damp: Stir in a pinch of ground ginger before blending.

If the weather is dry: Stir in a teaspoon of lemon juice before blending.

This is the perfect potion to sip when experiencing winter flu. It nourishes and hydrates the body without disrupting digestion.

4 carrots, sliced
4 cups water

1 teaspoon dried peppermint,
   or 1 peppermint tea bag

In a medium saucepan, combine all of the ingredients and bring to a boil. Reduce the heat to medium-low, cover loosely, and simmer until the carrots are very tender, about 15 minutes. If you're using a tea bag, discard it now. Blend or process the mixture until it is very smooth. Sip warm.

MAKES 4 SERVINGS; 30 CALORIES PER SERVING; NO ADDED FAT.

the cider cure

A doctor in Missouri told me that cider vinegar is antiseptic, and that those who imbibe it regularly escape winter flu and colds. In addition, for those who feel they are just "coming down" with something, drinking 1 cup of this brew every hour may subdue symptoms.

If the weather is damp: Drink the brew as is.

If the weather is dry: Stir in a teaspoon of honey before drinking.

1 cup hot water   **2 tablespoons cider vinegar**

Combine the water and cider in a mug and sip.

MAKES 1 SERVING; ABOUT 1 CALORIE; NO ADDED FAT.

sinus-soothing nasturtium tea

The peppery-tasting leaves in this Peruvian infusion help soothe a congested face and head. I learned about it from a Peruvian chef who, in his native land, drank the brew, and chewed raw nasturtium leaves to keep his sinuses clear.

If the weather is damp: Use 7 nasturtium leaves instead of 5.

If the weather is dry: Swirl in honey to taste, before drinking.

5 fresh nasturtium leaves   **1 cup hot water**

Soak the leaves in the water, covered, for about 10 minutes. Discard the leaves and sip the tea.

MAKES 1 SERVING; ABOUT 3 CALORIES; NO ADDED FAT.

decongesting syrup

If the weather is damp:
Take the syrup as is.

If the weather is dry: Swirl
I teaspoon lemon juice
into the tea or hot water,
before drinking.

This potent potion helps break up congestion in the lungs. It's a good alternative cough syrup for people who react to the artificial colors and flavors in some commercial syrups.

1 onion, finely chopped   **About 1¼ cups honey**

Put the onion in a shallow bowl and pour on the honey to cover. Cover the bowl with plastic wrap and let it sit at room temperature for about 8 hours, or overnight. Discard the onion and bottle the syrup. Swirl 1 tablespoon of the syrup in tea or hot water, 3 times a day.

MAKES ABOUT 16 TABLESPOONS; 65 CALORIES PER TABLESPOON; NO ADDED FAT.

deep spirits tea

If the weather is damp:
Add I star anise to the tea
before steeping.

If the weather is dry: Add
I teaspoon fennel seeds to
the tea before steeping.

Try this aromatic tea as a tonic when you're chilled, or when your mood is low. A Jamaican herbalist told me that cloves are an aphrodisiac, so you may wish to save a cup of tea for your sweetheart.

1 tablespoon cardamom pods   **2 cups hot water**
1 tablespoon black peppercorns   **2 cups orange juice, warmed**
1 tablespoon cloves

Combine all of the ingredients in a teapot, cover, and steep for 5 minutes. Discard the spices and sip.

MAKES 4 SERVINGS; 50 CALORIES PER SERVING; NO ADDED FAT.

japanese-style warming tonic

Try this quick and easy soup when you're dispirited and drained, to help warm and balance your body and mind. It's particularly useful in the late afternoon—take the tonic to work in a Thermos for a late-day rejuvenation.

If the weather is damp: Add a dash of soy sauce before sipping.

1 tablespoon finely grated radish   1 cup water
1 tablespoon finely grated carrot

If the weather is dry: Add a dash of lemon juice before sipping.

Combine all of the ingredients in a mug and sip. When you've finished the liquid, munch on the vegetables.

MAKES 1 SERVING; 25 CALORIES PER SERVING; NO ADDED FAT.

restful winter tea

The herbs that perfume this beverage—lemon verbena, chamomile, and lemon balm—contain aromatic compounds that help relax the mind and body.

If the weather is damp: Add a slice of fresh gingerroot before steeping.

½ teaspoon dried lemon balm   ½ teaspoon dried chamomile
½ teaspoon dried lemon verbena   1 cup pink grapefruit juice, warmed

If the weather is dry: Add 5 raisins before steeping.

Steep the herbs in the warmed juice, covered, for 4 minutes. Then discard the herbs and sip the tea.

MAKES 1 SERVING; 95 CALORIES PER SERVING; NO ADDED FAT.

rejuvenating winter tonic

If the weather is damp:
Garnish with minced
scallion to taste.

Miso, or fermented bean paste, helps enhance the entire body by strengthening the digestive system. The slightly salty flavor of this brew will help balance those who feel overly chilled and exhausted.

If the weather is dry:
Garnish with finely grated
carrot to taste.

½ to 1 teaspoon miso, any type   1 cup hot vegetable stock or water

Stir the miso into the stock and sip.

MAKES 1 SERVING; 25 CALORIES PER SERVING; NO ADDED FAT.

soothing winter foods

Chinese and Ayurvedic Indian healers note that with winter's shorter daylight hours and cooler temperatures, the body tends to contract. Think of what you do when you're cold—you clench your fists, scrunch up your shoulders, perhaps lock your jaw to keep your teeth from chattering. You contract your body in an attempt to conserve warmth. But since constantly tensed muscles are not conducive to a restful state of being, eating warming foods is recommended. Baking, stewing, braising, and other such long-cooking methods encourage a soothing warmth. Densely fleshed root vegetables such as carrots, parsnips, beets, sweet potatoes, and white potatoes, as well as warming whole-grain breads and buckwheat, can help balance the body and mind during the winter season. In addition, such heat-producing herbs and spices as garlic, onion, rosemary, and thyme can increase circulation, providing internal heat during this time of long, restful nights and short days.

MORE INTERESTING DATES IN JANUARY

January 7—Grey-Black Horse Ceremony in Japan, where those who eat rice porridge with ginger are said to escape ill luck for the entire year. January 21 (approximate)—The sun moves into the zodiac sign of Aquarius, the Water Bearer, symbolizing idealism. January (date floats)—Feast of the Kitchen God in China. In many Chinese kitchens, photos of the Kitchen God are hung over the stove. On this day, cooks take the photos down and burn them so the Kitchen God can ascend to heaven in a cloud of celestial smoke and deliver a good report on the cook. Those who participate in this ceremony give the house cook a break and dine out on this day. January 31—The Eve of Imbolic, an ancient Celtic holiday announcing spring's approach. As daylight increases, experiment with the holiday's intent by looking for hints of green sprouting from beneath the snow.

carrots
the stomach settler

A doctor in England told me that the best remedy for cranky digestion—particularly diarrhea and colitis—is cooked and pureed carrot diluted with an equal amount of hot water. (See Carrot-Peppermint Stomach Soother, page 8.) He claims that the pectin in the cooked carrots helps relax the digestive system, enabling it to rebalance itself and absorb nutrients. Proponents of the remedy say it is paramount when suffering from digestive upsets due to winter flu, and all manner of holiday overindulgences. Moreover, a female patron of the "carrot cure" told me it helps her with the kind of indigestion and headache that comes from drinking coffee that is overroasted or too acidic.

Carrots also soothe the skin and upper respiratory tract, due to the abundance of beta carotene they contain. One raw carrot, about 35 calories, offers over 200 percent of the Recommended Daily Allowance (RDA) for beta carotene. Note that peeling carrots will merely deprive you of the vegetables' weight—there is no extra nutrition in the skin.

carrots in captivity

Store carrots and apples separately. As apples ripen they give off ethylene, a gas that can make carrots taste bitter.

quick cooking tip for carrots

Peel older, drier-skinned carrots easily by using a swivel-bladed peeler (not a stationary blade). Young, tender specimens don't need peeling. Grate raw carrots into green salads to add color and nutrients; pack raw carrot sticks in plastic bags to snack on throughout the day and to take on airplane trips; for subtle sweetness add sliced carrots to simmering winter soups and stews, using one carrot per serving.

carrots with lemon-pepper dressing

The jalapeño in this recipe helps to increase circulation in the body, making the dish a good energizer for dreary winter days. In addition, the lemon is a gentle but effective "head opener" if you're feeling stuffy.

1 pound carrots, julienned
1 jalapeño pepper, seeded and
   minced
Juice of 2 lemons

1 teaspoon honey
½ teaspoon coriander seed, crushed
Pinch of sea salt

If the weather is damp: Add freshly ground pepper to the dressing before tossing with the carrots.

If the weather is dry: Serve the carrots as a salad on a bed of crisp greens.

Blanch the carrots in boiling water for about 1 minute, then drain and pat dry. In a medium bowl, toss the carrots with the jalapeño. In a small bowl, combine the lemon juice, honey, coriander seed, and salt. Pour it over the carrots and toss about 30 times. Serve at room temperature as a side dish or snack.

MAKES 4 SERVINGS; 93 CALORIES PER SERVING; NO ADDED FAT.

carrots with orange-soy marinade

If the weather is damp: Add 1 or 2 cloves of sliced garlic to the carrots and leeks when blanching.

If the weather is dry: Add a 2-inch ribbon of lemon peel to the marinade.

Orange is refreshing and hydrating in winter, especially if you've been in dry, overheated spaces. Make these citrus-scented "pickles" ahead and enjoy them to help banish winter fatigue.

1 pound carrots, peeled and
  sliced vertically

1 leek, topped, tailed, and thinly
  sliced

Juice of 2 oranges

2 teaspoons soy sauce or
  reduced-sodium soy sauce

1 teaspoon hot pepper sauce

1 teaspoon canola oil

1 to 2 cups rice vinegar, or to cover

1 teaspoon whole peppercorns

Blanch the carrots and leek in boiling water for about 30 seconds, then drain and arrange them in a shallow glass dish. Add the remaining ingredients, mix well, and cover. Let the carrots marinate, refrigerated, for at least an hour before enjoying as a snack or garnish. They will keep, covered and refrigerated in their marinade, for about a week.

MAKES 6 SERVINGS; 70 CALORIES PER SERVING; 1/2 GRAM OF FAT; 6 PERCENT OF CALORIES FROM FAT.

chunky carrots with garlic

Garlic contains sulfur compounds that can help rejuvenate a winter-worn body. It is also a good tonic for sluggish winter digestion.

1 pound carrots, cut into
   3/4-inch chunks
Juice of 1 lemon
1 teaspoon olive oil
1 tablespoon balsamic vinegar

3 cloves garlic, mashed through
   a press
2 scallions, minced
Pinch of sea salt

Steam the carrots over boiling water until they're tender, about 8 minutes.

Meanwhile, in a medium bowl, whisk together the remaining ingredients. Pat the carrots dry, toss them with the lemon mixture, and serve warm as a side dish.

MAKES 4 SERVINGS; 103 CALORIES PER SERVING; 1 GRAM OF FAT; 9 PERCENT OF CALORIES FROM FAT.

If the weather is damp: Grind on fresh black pepper before serving.

If the weather is dry: Add a tablespoon minced fresh parsley when tossing the carrots with the lemon mixture, and serve the dish at room temperature or slightly chilled.

carrot-garlic-miso pickles

In Japan, this fortifying condiment is eaten in the winter months to help nourish the body deeply.

1 cup thinly sliced carrots
12 cloves garlic, peeled and thinly
   sliced

1 cup any variety of miso (available
   at natural food stores and Asian
   markets)

Combine all of the ingredients in a glass jar, making sure all of the carrot and garlic are covered with miso. Cover the jar and refrigerate for at least 2 weeks. The miso "pickles" the carrot and garlic, and will keep for up to a year. To eat, remove a garlic slice and several carrots from the jar, lightly brushing off the clinging miso before enjoying as a condiment to rice or noodle dishes.

MAKES 12 CONDIMENT SERVINGS; 25 CALORIES PER SERVING; NO ADDED FAT.

If the weather is damp: Splash the pickles with hot pepper sauce before serving.

If the weather is dry: Serve as an accompaniment to steamed or sweet potatoes.

brown rice with fragrant vegetables

If the weather is damp: Serve with a side dish of roasted onions or other roasted vegetables.

If the weather is dry: Serve with a side dish of steamed vegetables.

Carrots add a delicate sweetness to this fortifying winter entrée. Pack it to take to work, where the B vitamins in the brown rice will help to soothe your nerves.

1 tablespoon olive oil

2 cloves garlic, finely minced

1 shallot, finely minced

2 leeks, topped, tailed, and chopped

4 artichoke hearts (frozen or
    canned), chopped

1 cup grated carrots

2 cups cooked brown rice

2 tablespoons freshly grated Romano
    or soy cheese

Heat a large sauté pan on medium-high, then add the olive oil. When the oil is warm, add the garlic, shallot, leeks, artichokes, and carrots, and sauté until they're tender, about 4 minutes. Add the rice and continue to sauté until the rice is warm, about 2 minutes more. Stir in the cheese and serve warm for lunch or dinner.

MAKES 4 SERVINGS; 200 CALORIES PER SERVING; 5 GRAMS OF FAT; 22 PERCENT OF CALORIES FROM FAT.

italian rice with carrot, leek, and saffron

This entrée is made with Italian arborio rice. Famous for its short grains, arborio offers a creamy texture without having to add actual cream. This is a cold-weather plus, when a heavier-textured yet low-fat dish may be what you're craving.

5 cups vegetable stock

2 teaspoons olive oil

1 leek, topped, tailed, and chopped

1½ cups uncooked arborio rice
   (available at specialty stores and
   many supermarkets)

½ teaspoon saffron threads

1 carrot, grated

2 tablespoons freshly grated
   Parmesan or soy cheese

2 scallions, minced

If the weather is damp: Sprinkle in a pinch of cayenne when adding the cheese.

If the weather is dry: Serve with a side of steamed greens, such as collards or kale, dressed with lemon juice and olive oil.

Pour the vegetable stock into a large saucepan and warm it on low heat.

Meanwhile, heat a large frying pan and add the olive oil. Toss in the leek and rice and sauté until fragrant, about 3 minutes.

Ladle in enough stock just to cover the rice, add the saffron, and simmer gently, using a rubber spatula to stir frequently until the rice has absorbed all of the stock. Then add another cup of stock and continue to stir and simmer. Don't rush. If the fire is too hot, the rice won't be creamy. Keep adding stock by the cup until all 5 cups have been absorbed, a process which should take about 25 minutes. Immediately toss in the grated carrot, cheese, and scallions; combine well; and serve warm or at room temperature as a lunch or dinner entrée.

MAKES 4 SERVINGS; 321 CALORIES PER SERVING; 3 GRAMS OF FAT; 9 PERCENT OF CALORIES FROM FAT.

vegetable soup with orzo

If the weather is damp: Swirl in a spoonful of spicy salsa before serving.

If the weather is dry: Serve chilled, fresh oranges for dessert.

The combination of sage and thyme helps to enliven the flavor of this soup, and also provides soothing aromatics that help unclog a stuffy winter head.

1 tablespoon olive oil
1 onion, chopped
1 leek, topped, tailed, and chopped
2 cloves garlic, minced
1 bay leaf
2 medium carrots, chopped
2 celery stalks, chopped
10 medium-sized fresh mushrooms, chopped
1 large potato, chopped

1 large sweet potato, chopped
1½ quarts vegetable stock
Juice of 1 lemon
1 teaspoon minced fresh sage
1 teaspoon minced fresh thyme
2 tomatoes, chopped (canned may be used)
¼ cup raw orzo pasta
Pinch of sea salt, or to taste
¼ cup minced fresh parsley

Heat a large soup pot on medium-high, then add the oil. Add the onion, leek, garlic, and bay leaf and sauté until they're fragrant and just soft, about 5 minutes. Add the carrots, celery, mushrooms, potato, and sweet potato and sauté for 5 minutes more. Add the stock, lemon juice, sage, and thyme and bring to a boil. Reduce the heat to a simmer, cover loosely, and continue to simmer until the vegetables are tender, about 35 minutes. Stir and smell occasionally.

Uncover the soup and bring it to a boil. Add the tomatoes, orzo, and salt and continue to boil, uncovered, until the orzo is tender, about 10 minutes. Serve the soup warm, garnished with the parsley, as a lunch or dinner entrée.

MAKES ABOUT 2 QUARTS, OR EIGHT 1-CUP SERVINGS; 120 CALORIES PER SERVING; 2 GRAMS OF FAT; 15 PERCENT OF CALORIES FROM FAT.

carrot soup with fresh ginger

In Vietnam, gingerroot is added to winter soups to warm the body. The garlic also contributes warmth, as it helps increase circulation.

5 carrots, chopped
1 potato, peeled and chopped
1 tablespoon minced fresh gingerroot

2 cloves garlic, sliced
2 cups soy or skim milk
Pinch of sea salt

Steam the carrots, potato, gingerroot, and garlic over boiling water until they're tender, about 12 minutes. Meanwhile, in a small saucepan, heat the milk gently; don't boil.

When the vegetables are tender, puree them (including the ginger and garlic) in a food processor or blender; then stir, along with the salt, into the waiting warmed milk. Serve warm as a lunch or dinner entrée.

MAKES 4 SERVINGS; 135 CALORIES PER SERVING; NO ADDED FAT.

If the weather is damp: When adding the pureed vegetables to the warmed milk, stir in hot pepper sauce to taste.

If the weather is dry: Stir in a tablespoon fresh lime juice to the warmed soup before serving.

carrot-miso soup

I like this soup as a quick winter restorative. The sweet carrots contrast deliciously with the slightly salty miso, making an agreeable and interestingly wholesome flavor.

4 cups vegetable stock
5 carrots, sliced
1 onion, sliced

¼ cup any kind of miso (available at natural food stores and Asian markets)
3 scallions, minced

In a medium saucepan, combine the stock, carrots, and onion and bring to a boil. Reduce the heat to medium-low, cover loosely, and simmer until the carrots are tender, 12 to 15 minutes. Put the miso in a small strainer and submerge it in the soup. Use a spoon to rub the miso through the strainer, diffusing it into the soup. Remove the soup from the heat, add the scallions, and serve with lunch or dinner, or as a fortifying snack.

MAKES 4 SERVINGS; 105 CALORIES PER SERVING; .75 GRAM OF FAT; 7 PERCENT OF CALORIES FROM FAT.

If the weather is damp: Add 1 or 2 cloves of minced garlic to the soup before simmering.

If the weather is dry: Add ¼ cup diced water chestnuts to the soup before simmering.

carrot bread with dill and chives

If the weather is damp:
Toast slices before
enjoying.

If the weather is dry:
Spread slices with all-fruit
apricot preserves before
enjoying.

A slice of this tasty bread may well be an antidote to winter stress. In addition to the carrots' calming digestive effects, this loaf contains the stomach-soothing herb dillweed.

2 tablespoons active dry yeast
2¼ cups warm vegetable stock or
    water
1 tablespoon honey
1 tablespoon olive oil
3 carrots, sliced, steamed, and
    pureed

¼ cup minced fresh chives
2 tablespoons minced fresh dillweed
1 teaspoon fine sea salt
About 3 cups unbleached flour
About 3 cups whole wheat bread
    flour

Preheat the oven to 350°F. Lightly oil a 9 × 5-inch loaf pan.

In a bowl, dissolve the yeast in ½ cup of the warm stock by stirring well with a fork. Then stir in the honey. When the yeast is beginning to bubble, add the remaining stock. Stir in the oil, pureed carrots, chives, dill, and salt. Then work in about 1½ cups of each of the flours (a total of 3 cups) until you have a loose dough. Transfer the loose dough to a counter and knead in enough of the remaining flours to make a dough that's firm enough to handle. Then knead the dough for about 7 minutes.

Set the kneaded dough in a lightly oiled bowl, turning it once so all surfaces are touched with oil. Cover the bowl with plastic wrap and set it in a warm place until the dough has doubled in size, about 45 minutes. Use your fist to punch down the dough, then divide the dough into 2 pieces. Knead each piece lightly until it is smooth; then set each piece into the prepared pans. Cover each pan with plastic wrap and let the loaves rise until nearly doubled in size, about 30 minutes.

Bake the loaves for about 35 minutes, or until the bread is lightly browned and sounds hollow when tapped. Let the loaves cool before slicing. Serve with winter soups, or as sandwich bread.

MAKES 2 LOAVES, OR 24 THICK SLICES; 117 CALORIES PER SLICE; ½ GRAM OF FAT; 7 PERCENT OF CALORIES FROM FAT.

parsnips
love your lungs

At an East Hampton, New York, Thanksgiving party I sat down next to a lively elderly woman from Ireland. After offering me half her beer, she went on to tell how Irish women use mashed, cooked parsnips to treat lingering winter coughs and consumption. Parsnips help heal the lungs and strengthen the whole body, she claimed, and young people today would do well to eat them regularly in cold weather.

One way parsnips may work is that they contain a smooth, soothing pectin that helps to relax the lungs. In addition, parsnips offer digestion-strengthening insoluble fiber. Half a cup of cooked parsnips contains about 65 calories and virtually no fat. And the high fiber content may make you feel fuller faster, thus aiding weight loss.

picking parsnips

Parsnips look like cream-colored carrots. Choose small- to medium-sized ones with smooth skin. Larger parsnips taste fine, but their texture can be woody.

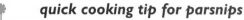

✳ quick cooking tip for parsnips

Try substituting parsnips for half the carrots in such recipes as breads, cakes, side dishes, and soups. Or steam (for about ten minutes, or until tender) and mash parsnips, and serve them as you would mashed potatoes.

parsnips with aromatic herbs

If the weather is damp:
Add a splash of hot pepper
sauce when sautéing the
herbs.

If the weather is dry:
Double the lemon juice to
2 teaspoons.

The uplifting combination of garlic, basil, and scallion makes this a perfect dish for the winter-worn. Moreover, the fragrant parsnips may subdue a craving for sweets, without adding fat and refined sugar.

1 pound parsnips, cut into 1-inch
  chunks
1 teaspoon olive oil
1 scallion, minced
1 clove garlic, minced

1 tablespoon minced fresh basil
Pinch of sea salt
Freshly ground black pepper
1 teaspoon lemon juice

Steam the parsnips over boiling water until they're just tender, 10 to 12 minutes. Drain and pat dry.

Meanwhile, heat a medium sauté pan on medium-high heat and add the oil. Add the remaining ingredients, and sauté for 1 minute. Add the steamed parsnips and heat through, stirring constantly, for 1 to 2 minutes. Serve warm as a side dish for lunch or dinner.

MAKES 4 SERVINGS; 80 CALORIES PER SERVING; 1 GRAM OF FAT; 12 PERCENT OF CALORIES FROM FAT.

garlic-mashed parsnips

Since winter weather may aggravate aches and pains due to arthritis, people who are susceptible to this condition may wish to switch from mashed potatoes to mashed parsnips. Potatoes contain a compound called "solanine," which may worsen arthritis.

1 pound parsnips, peeled and chopped	½ cup plain nonfat yogurt or soy yogurt
6 cloves garlic, peeled and sliced	Pinch of sea salt
1 teaspoon olive oil	3 tablespoons minced fresh parsley

Steam the parsnips and garlic over boiling water until they're very tender, 12 to 14 minutes. Drain and pat dry. Tip the parsnips and garlic into a medium bowl and begin to mash, adding the olive oil, yogurt, salt, and parsley as you go. Serve warm as a lunch or dinner side dish.

MAKES 4 SERVINGS; 101 CALORIES PER SERVING; 1 GRAM OF FAT; 9 PERCENT OF CALORIES FROM FAT.

If the weather is damp: Add freshly ground pepper when mashing the parsnips.

If the weather is dry: Mash in extra yogurt, or a couple of tablespoons of steaming water, to make a moister dish.

warm parsnip salad with lemon-rosemary dressing

If the weather is damp:
Add 1 tablespoon minced
fresh chives when tossing
to combine.

―――――

If the weather is dry: Serve
on a bed of crisp greens.

Winter temperature changes—going from cold outside to warm inside—can sometimes trigger a headache. This rosemary-scented recipe may help, since the herb contains a compound called "rosmaricine" that can ease head pain.

¾ pound parsnips, cut into ½-inch slices

¼ pound carrots, cut into ½-inch slices

2 teaspoons minced fresh rosemary, or 1 teaspoon dried

2 tablespoons lemon juice

1 tablespoon orange juice

½ teaspoon Dijon-style mustard

2 teaspoons olive oil

Steam the parsnips and carrots over boiling water until they're just tender, about 12 minutes. Drain, pat dry, and slip them into a medium bowl.

In a small bowl, whisk together the rosemary, lemon and orange juices, mustard, and oil. Pour over the parsnips and carrots and toss well to combine. Serve warm as an appetizer, salad, or side dish.

MAKES 4 SERVINGS; 105 CALORIES PER SERVING; 2 GRAMS OF FAT; 16 PERCENT OF CALORIES FROM FAT.

leek-braised parsnips

Perfumed with tarragon, this dish tones a sluggish winter digestive system. Tarragon is an especially refreshing tonic for those who have overindulged in fatty foods.

If the weather is damp: Add a dried hot pepper to the stock before braising.

2 cups vegetable stock
1 bay leaf
2 leeks, topped, tailed, and sliced
1 clove garlic, minced
1 pound parsnips, sliced

Juice of 1 lemon
2 teaspoons olive oil
1 teaspoon minced fresh tarragon,
   or ½ teaspoon dried
Pinch of sea salt

If the weather is dry: Serve the dish on a nest of steamed kale or collards.

In a large frying pan, heat the stock on high. When it begins to simmer, add the bay leaf, leeks, garlic, and parsnips. Cover loosely and continue to simmer until the parsnips are tender, about 9 minutes. Remove the leeks and parsnips from the braising stock with a slotted spoon and arrange them in a serving bowl.

In a small bowl, combine the lemon juice, olive oil, tarragon, and salt. Sprinkle the mixture over the parsnips and serve warm as a first course or side dish.

MAKES 4 SERVINGS; 140 CALORIES PER SERVING; 2 GRAMS OF FAT; 14 PERCENT OF CALORIES FROM FAT.

warm parsnip salad with mustard sauce

If the weather is damp: Sprinkle with freshly ground pepper before serving.

If the weather is dry: Add 1 tomato, chopped (canned may be used), when tossing the parsnips with the dressing.

Mustard is a good source of magnesium, a mineral whose absence in the body is linked to irritability caused by PMS and menopause. Winter may aggravate these problems, since short daylight hours are linked to bad moods in both men and women.

1 pound parsnips, sliced	1 tablespoon balsamic vinegar
3 cups water	1 tablespoon Dijon-style mustard
1 tablespoon olive oil	1 tablespoon minced fresh chives

Add the parsnips to about 3 cups of boiling water and blanch until they're just beginning to soften, about 3 minutes. Drain and pat dry.

In a small bowl, whisk together the oil, vinegar, mustard, and chives. Toss with the parsnips and serve warm as a first course or side dish.

MAKES 4 SERVINGS; 120 CALORIES PER SERVING; 3.5 GRAMS OF FAT; 26 PERCENT OF CALORIES FROM FAT.

fresh parsnip salad with beets and carrots

If the weather is damp: Serve with toasted whole wheat pita bread.

If the weather is dry: Substitute 1 tablespoon lemon juice for the cider vinegar.

When you're parched from overheated winter spaces, here's a hydrating and rejuvenating repast.

⅓ pound parsnips, coarsely grated	1 tablespoon cider vinegar
⅓ pound carrots, coarsely grated	1 tablespoon balsamic vinegar
⅓ pound golden beets, coarsely grated	2 teaspoons olive oil
	Pinch of sea salt

In a medium bowl, combine the parsnips, carrots, and beets. In a small bowl, combine the vinegars, oil, and salt, and pour over the vegetables. Toss well to combine and serve at room temperature as a first course or side dish.

MAKES 4 SERVINGS; 112 CALORIES PER SERVING; 2 GRAMS OF FAT; 15 PERCENT OF CALORIES FROM FAT.

parsnips with garlic and whole wheat crumbs

Often in winter the most comforting and restful foods are the simplest, which certainly is the case with this wholesome and nourishing repast.

1 pound parsnips, sliced

2 teaspoons olive oil

2 cloves garlic, minced

2 slices whole wheat bread, rubbed
   into crumbs

2 tablespoons minced fresh basil

Pinch of sea salt

If the weather is damp: Sprinkle with freshly grated nutmeg before serving.

If the weather is dry: Toss with 2 cups just-cooked pasta and serve warm.

Steam the parsnips over boiling water until they're tender, 10 to 12 minutes. Drain and pat dry.

Preheat a sauté pan, then heat the olive oil on medium-high and add the garlic, crumbs, basil, and salt. Sauté until the ingredients are fragrant and heated through, about 2 minutes. Add the parsnips and stir to combine. Serve warm as a side dish for lunch or dinner.

MAKES 4 SERVINGS; 140 CALORIES PER SERVING; 2 GRAMS OF FAT; 14 PERCENT OF CALORIES FROM FAT.

curried parsnip puree

If the weather is damp: Add a splash of hot pepper sauce to the curry mixture.

If the weather is dry: Add I teaspoon lemon juice to the curry mixture.

Curry powder contains turmeric, a spice that Ayurvedic Indian herbalists prescribe to counteract winter irritability and promote a peaceful disposition.

1 pound parsnips, sliced
2 teaspoons olive oil

1 teaspoon curry powder, or to taste
1 shallot, minced

Simmer the sliced parsnips in water to cover until tender, about 10 minutes. Drain the parsnips and pat them dry. Then place them in a food processor or blender and puree.

Heat a sauté pan on medium-high and warm the oil. Add the curry powder and shallot and sauté until the shallot begins to brown and the curry is fragrant, about 4 minutes. Use a rubber spatula to scrape the curry mixture into the parsnips and combine well. Serve warm as a side dish for lunch or dinner.

MAKES 4 SERVINGS; 75 CALORIES PER SERVING; 2 GRAMS OF FAT; 27 PERCENT OF CALORIES FROM FAT.

parsnip soup with garlic

This soup, based on an ancient Japanese healing formula, helps to restore the body and rebalance it after a long winter's day. The nettle and parsley each contain a "multivitamin" of nourishing nutrients, and the garlic energizes the body and mind by increasing circulation.

1 quart water
2 tablespoons dried nettle or dried
   parsley (nettle is available at herb
   shops and natural food stores)
1 large bulb garlic, peeled and
   chopped

4 parsnips, chopped
4 teaspoons any kind of miso
   (available at natural food stores
   and Asian markets)

If the weather is damp: Add hot pepper sauce to taste to each serving.

If the weather is dry: Add lemon juice to taste to each serving.

In a large soup pot, combine the water, nettle, garlic, and parsnips and bring to a boil. Reduce the heat to medium, cover loosely, and simmer until the parsnips are very tender, about 15 minutes.

Using a slotted spoon, remove the garlic and parsnips and puree them in a blender or food processor. Return them to the soup. Scoop the miso into a strainer, submerge it in the soup, and use a spoon to rub through the strainer, diffusing it into the soup. Remove the soup from the heat, stir well, and serve warm with a sandwich for lunch, or as a first course for dinner.

MAKES 4 SERVINGS; 70 CALORIES PER SERVING; TRACE OF FAT.

parsnip soup with wild rice and fresh thyme

If the weather is damp:
Add cayenne to taste
before serving.

If the weather is dry: Serve
with a crisp green salad.

Enjoy this soup as a winter evening tonic when you feel worn. The thyme contains aromatic, anti-infective compounds that help stave off colds and flu.

1 tablespoon olive oil
1 onion, chopped
1 leek, chopped
1 pound parsnips, finely chopped
1 bay leaf
3 cloves garlic, minced

4 cups vegetable stock
¼ cup uncooked wild rice
1 tablespoon minced fresh thyme, or
  1½ teaspoons dried
Pinch of sea salt

Heat a large soup pot over medium heat and warm the oil. Add the onion, leek, parsnips, bay leaf, and garlic. Sauté until the vegetables are fragrant and slightly soft, about 8 minutes.

Add the stock, rice, thyme, and salt and bring the soup to a boil. Reduce the heat to medium-low, cover loosely, and continue to simmer for about an hour. Serve warm for lunch with a sandwich, or as a first course for dinner.

MAKES 4 SERVINGS; 150 CALORIES PER SERVING; 5 GRAMS OF FAT; 30 PERCENT OF CALORIES FROM FAT.

beets
the wonder root

A rosy-cheeked Mennonite woman at a farmers' market near Lancaster, Pennsylvania, told me that eating beets is the secret to fighting winter fatigue. They're a good source of the energizing mineral iron, she said, and she and the women in her family eat them, pickled or boiled, nearly every winter day.

On the nutritional charts, one serving of cooked beets (about half a cup) contains half a gram of iron. The Recommended Daily Allowance (RDA) for iron is approximately 18 milligrams, which may not seem like a lot until you factor in the knowledge that vitamin C helps the body absorb iron, and beets contain vitamin C, too. By contrast, half a cup of cooked soybeans contains about 8 grams of iron but no vitamin C, so the iron from the beans may not be absorbed by the body as well as the iron from the beets.

Another way that beets may stave off winter fatigue is that they contain nearly half the RDA for folate, a nutrient whose absence in the diet is associated with low energy and depression.

the shocking truth

Some people who eat lots of beets are shocked to find that their urine turns red. This benign condition is called "beeturia," and while it is disconcerting, it is only temporary.

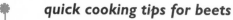

quick cooking tips for beets

To get these roots into your diet, grate raw beets into salads. Peel, slice, and steam beets until tender (about eight minutes) and toss with fresh orange sections for a refreshing salad. Stir half a cup of steamed, pureed beets into two cups of hot soup to thicken without cream or butter.

warm beets with tarragon and mustard

If the weather is damp: Add a pinch of dried mustard when whisking in the prepared mustard.

If the weather is dry: Sprinkle the beets with 1 teaspoon lemon juice before drizzling on the sauce.

Ayurvedic Indian healers say that beets are calming and encourage a restful mood. The mustard, which flavors the recipe, helps also by offering nerve-soothing magnesium.

1 tablespoon olive oil or butter
1 tablespoon flour
½ cup vegetable stock
½ cup skim milk or soy milk
1 tablespoon Dijon-style mustard

1 tablespoon minced fresh chives
1 teaspoon minced fresh tarragon, or
    ½ teaspoon dried
8 beets, cooked and sliced

Heat the olive oil or butter in a small saucepan over medium heat and whisk in the flour. Stir constantly for 1 to 2 minutes. Remove the pan from the heat and whisk in the stock and milk. Return the pan to the heat and, whisking constantly, bring the sauce to a boil, continuing to boil for about 1 minute. Remove the sauce from the heat and stir in the mustard, chives, and tarragon. Arrange the beets on a platter and drizzle on the sauce. Serve warm as a side dish for lunch or dinner.

MAKES 4 SERVINGS; 80 CALORIES PER SERVING; 3.5 GRAMS OF FAT; 37 PERCENT OF CALORIES FROM FAT.

ginger-glazed beets

Spicy gingerroot increases circulation, thus helping the body to stay warm in winter. Its volatile oils also make ginger an excellent digestive tonic.

1 tablespoon canola oil or butter

1 teaspoon lemon juice

¼ cup all-fruit apricot jam

1 tablespoon gingerroot juice
(squeezed from ¼ cup grated
gingerroot)

Pinch of sea salt

1 pound beets, sliced and cooked

If the weather is damp: Add a pinch of freshly grated nutmeg to the glaze.

If the weather is dry: Increase the lemon juice to 2 teaspoons.

In a medium saucepan, combine the oil or butter, the lemon juice, jam, ginger, and salt and bring to a boil. Reduce the heat to low and simmer, stirring frequently, until the glaze is fragrant and slightly thick, about 4 minutes. Add the beets and gently toss, heating through for about 1 minute. Serve warm as a side dish for lunch or dinner.

MAKES 4 SERVINGS; 120 CALORIES PER SERVING; 3.5 GRAMS OF FAT; 27 PERCENT OF CALORIES FROM FAT.

beets braised in bay, cinnamon, and honey

German herbalists prescribe daily doses of cinnamon to strengthen weak winter digestion. The essential oils it contains soothe stomach spasms, and tone the entire digestive system.

1 pound beets, quartered

One 2-inch stick of cinnamon

1 bay leaf

2 tablespoons honey

2 cups brewed orange-flavored
herbal tea

Pinch of sea salt

If the weather is damp: Add 5 whole peppercorns to the braising liquid.

If the weather is dry: After removing the cooked beets from the braising liquid, bring the liquid to a boil and continue to boil until it has been reduced by half. (If not much liquid is left, add ½ cup more of tea or water.) Strain and pour over the beets before serving.

In a medium saucepan, combine all of the ingredients and bring to a boil. Reduce the heat, cover loosely, and simmer until the beets are fragrant and tender, 15 to 20 minutes. Remove the beets from the braising liquid and serve warm as a side dish for lunch or dinner.

MAKES 4 SERVINGS; 80 CALORIES PER SERVING; NO ADDED FAT.

sautéed beet greens with garlic and ginger

If the weather is damp:
Use 2 cloves of garlic.

If the weather is dry:
Sprinkle with crumbled
feta cheese before serving.

If you want two vegetables for the price of one, when shopping for beetroots, look for those with crisp greens attached. The greens can be cooked like spinach, kale, and collards, and are a good source of the mood-soothing mineral magnesium.

1 teaspoon olive oil	3 cups sliced beet greens
1 clove garlic, minced	¼ cup vegetable stock
½ teaspoon finely minced	Pinch of sea salt
gingerroot	2 scallions, minced

Preheat a large sauté pan on medium-high and add the oil. When the oil is warm, add the garlic, ginger, greens, stock, and salt, and sauté until the liquid has nearly evaporated and the greens are just wilted, 3 to 4 minutes. Sprinkle with the scallions and serve warm as a side dish for lunch or dinner.

MAKES 4 SERVINGS; 65 CALORIES PER SERVING; 1 GRAM OF FAT; 18 PERCENT OF CALORIES FROM FAT.

beet greens with potatoes and rosemary

If the weather is damp:
Serve the greens with
toasted whole wheat pita
bread.

If the weather is dry:
Sprinkle on freshly grated
Parmesan cheese before
serving.

For an antidote to winter constipation, try beet greens. They contain insoluble fiber and make a tasty high-fiber alternative to bran cereals.

2 teaspoons olive oil	2 medium potatoes, cubed and
2 cloves garlic, minced	steamed
1 teaspoon minced fresh rosemary,	2 cups chopped beet greens
or ½ teaspoon dried	Pinch of sea salt

Preheat a sauté pan on medium-high and add the oil. When the oil is warm, add all the remaining ingredients and toss well to combine. Sauté until the greens are wilted and the rosemary and garlic are fragrant, about 4 minutes. Serve warm as a side dish for lunch or dinner, or with an omelet for brunch.

MAKES 4 SERVINGS; 105 CALORIES PER SERVING; 2 GRAMS OF FAT; 17 PERCENT OF CALORIES FROM FAT.

sweet potato
sweet protection

One January 26, while eating pie made from mashed sweet potato and white beans, I learned about African numerology from a woman from the Ivory Coast. The pie was silky, and sweet with honey, but according to legend, the day was not. The number six, said the woman, can indicate chaos, and this day was double six (two times six), which means double chaos. It's always best to lie low on the twenty-sixth of each month, she said, but if you can't, you can opt for eating a slice of sweet potato pie to soothe and sweeten any tensions that may occur.

Sweet potatoes are a good choice any day of the month, especially in winter, since one tuber contains a huge amount—43,000 I.U.—of beta carotene, a nutrient that can help protect the lungs from disease and keep the skin and eyes healthy. One medium-sized sweet potato contains about 120 calories and virtually no fat, making it a nourishing winter food that won't contribute to weight gain.

sweet relations

Sweet potatoes are not related botanically to either white potatoes or yams. Yams are actually huge tubers that grow in such hot areas as parts of South America, New Guinea, and Africa. You can find yams, cut into large chunks and shrink-wrapped in Latino and African markets, and though yams are botanically different from sweet potatoes, they have a very similar taste and texture, and can be used interchangeably in recipes.

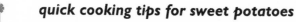

✳ quick cooking tips for sweet potatoes

Bake sweet potatoes as you would white potatoes and flavor them with minced scallion. Steam sweet potatoes (in chunks, for about twelve minutes, or until tender) and mash as you would white potatoes. Make a warm sweet potato salad instead of a white potato salad, for a sweeter winter day.

warm sweet potatoes with cinnamon and cloves

If the weather is damp: Add a pinch of ground ginger when mashing.

If the weather is dry: Add a pinch of finely grated fresh orange peel.

According to Ayurvedic Indian healers, cinnamon and cloves help warm the body, thanks to the stimulating volatile oils they contain.

2 large sweet potatoes, peeled and cubed

½ cup unsweetened applesauce

1 teaspoon orange juice

½ teaspoon ground cinnamon

¼ teaspoon ground cloves

Pinch of sea salt

Set the sweet potatoes in a medium saucepan and partially cover with water. Cover the pan and bring the water to a boil. Reduce the heat, cover loosely, and simmer until the sweet potatoes are tender, about 15 minutes. Drain and pat dry.

In a medium bowl, mash the sweet potatoes, adding the applesauce, orange juice, cinnamon, cloves, and salt as you go. Serve warm as a side dish for lunch or dinner.

MAKES 4 SERVINGS; 90 CALORIES PER SERVING; NO ADDED FAT.

baked sweet potatoes with apples and cinnamon

Aromatherapists say that the scent of cinnamon, such as that which perfumes this winter side dish, is a mild stimulant to the circulatory, heart, and nervous systems. Clinical studies also indicate that the aroma of cinnamon can be an aphrodisiac. The apples, too, are an apt tonic, containing soluble fiber to help regulate blood sugar and blood cholesterol levels.

2 sweet potatoes, sliced
2 tart apples, sliced
½ cup apple juice

1 bay leaf
½ teaspoon ground cinnamon
Pinch of sea salt

If the weather is damp: Add 1 teaspoon minced fresh gingerroot.

If the weather is dry: Add 2 lemon slices to the dish before baking.

Preheat the oven to 375°F.

In a medium-sized oven dish, combine all of the ingredients and cover. Bake until the sweet potatoes are tender, about 45 minutes. Serve warm as a side dish for lunch or dinner.

MAKES 4 SERVINGS; 105 CALORIES PER SERVING; NO ADDED FAT.

mashed sweet potatoes with orange and nutmeg

The smell of orange, aroma experts say, can be uplifting and help create a restful atmosphere.

3 sweet potatoes, peeled and cubed
2 carrots, sliced
¼ cup orange juice

¼ teaspoon finely grated orange rind
¼ teaspoon freshly grated nutmeg
Pinch of sea salt

If the weather is damp: Increase the nutmeg to ½ teaspoon.

If the weather is dry: Serve with orange slices for garnish; or scoop into hollowed-out orange skins and serve.

Steam the sweet potatoes and carrots over boiling water until they're tender, about 20 minutes. Tip them into a medium bowl along with the remaining ingredients and mash. Serve warm as a side dish for lunch or dinner.

MAKES 4 SERVINGS; 60 CALORIES PER SERVING; NO ADDED FAT.

sweet potato soup with lemongrass and scallion

If the weather is damp:
Increase the hot pepper
sauce to taste.

If the weather is dry:
Double the basil.

Lemongrass contains volatile oils that can help to soothe a stressed stomach. The basil, which also perfumes the recipe, is what herbalists call a "carminative," a substance that soothes digestion.

3 cups vegetable stock

2 teaspoons nam pla (available at Asian markets) or soy sauce

1 teaspoon hot pepper sauce

1 tablespoon minced fresh lemongrass, or 1½ teaspoons dried

1 sweet potato, diced

3 scallions, cut into julienne

1 tablespoon minced fresh basil

In a medium soup pot, combine the stock, nam pla or soy sauce, hot pepper sauce, lemongrass, and sweet potato and bring to a boil. Reduce the heat, cover loosely, and simmer until the soup is fragrant and the sweet potato is tender, about 20 minutes. Stir in the scallions and basil and serve warm with a salad for lunch, or as a first course for dinner.

MAKES 4 SERVINGS; 60 CALORIES PER SERVING; NO ADDED FAT.

creamy sweet potato–leek soup

The wisp of nutmeg in this silky soup is used by herbalists to treat cranky digestion after a stressful day.

2 sweet potatoes, peeled and
   chunked
2 leeks, topped, tailed, and chopped
1 onion, chopped
1 shallot, chopped

2 cups vegetable stock
Pinch of sea salt
¼ teaspoon freshly grated nutmeg
1 cup skim milk, whole milk, or soy
   milk, warmed

In a medium saucepan, combine the sweet potatoes, leeks, onion, shallot, stock, salt, and nutmeg and bring to a boil. Reduce the heat, cover loosely, and simmer until the sweet potatoes are very tender, about 25 minutes. Puree in a blender or food processor, adding the milk as you go. Serve warm as an entrée for lunch or dinner.

MAKES 4 SERVINGS; 160 CALORIES PER SERVING; NO ADDED FAT.

*If the weather is damp:
Add hot pepper sauce to
taste before simmering.*

*If the weather is dry:
Substitute 1 cup tomato
juice for 1 cup stock.*

spicy sweet potato soup

I sampled a soup like this in Zimbabwe, where squash, peanuts, garlic, and hot peppers serve to energize the mind and body gently.

1 cup vegetable stock
2 cloves garlic, minced
1 onion, minced
2 sweet potatoes, diced
1 celery stalk, minced
2 tablespoons peanut butter

1 teaspoon hot pepper sauce, or to
   taste
Pinch of sea salt
2 cups skim milk, soy milk, or whole
   milk, warmed

In a medium sauté pan, combine the stock, garlic, onion, sweet potatoes, and celery, and cook on high until the sweet potato is very tender, about 25 minutes. Puree in a food processor or blender adding the peanut butter, hot pepper sauce, salt, and milk as you go. Serve warm as an entrée for lunch or dinner.

MAKES 4 SERVINGS; 245 CALORIES PER SERVING; 4 GRAMS OF FAT; 15 PERCENT OF CALORIES FROM FAT.

*If the weather is damp:
Serve topped with
croutons.*

*If the weather is dry: Serve
topped with chopped fresh
or canned tomato.*

baked winter stew with fresh thyme

*If the weather is damp:
Serve the stew with a
crusty loaf of whole-grain
bread.*

*If the weather is dry: Serve
the stew with pepper-
mint tea.*

The winter vegetables in this hearty dish are made fragrant with thyme, an herb containing antiseptic properties that help fight winter colds and flu.

2 cloves garlic, minced

2 onions, chopped

2 sweet potatoes, chopped

4 carrots, chopped

1 teaspoon dried hot pepper flakes

3 cups vegetable stock or water

2 tablespoons minced fresh thyme,
   or 1 tablespoon dried

Pinch of sea salt

¼ cup minced fresh parsley

1 teaspoon olive oil

Preheat the oven to 350°F.

In a large casserole dish, combine the garlic, onions, sweet potatoes, carrots, hot pepper flakes, stock or water, thyme, and salt. Cover and bake until the vegetables are tender, about 45 minutes. For a thicker stew, remove the casserole cover for the last 15 minutes of baking. Swirl in the parsley and olive oil before serving warm as an entrée for brunch, lunch, or dinner.

MAKES 4 SERVINGS; 140 CALORIES PER SERVING; 1 GRAM OF FAT; 7 PERCENT OF CALORIES FROM FAT.

sweet potato soup with fennel

Fennel is what herbalists call an antispasmodic, a substance that soothes stressed digestion. Fennel is also a natural, mild diuretic—good news for those who feel bloated from eating salty foods.

2 teaspoons olive oil

2 cloves garlic, minced

1 leek, topped, tailed, and chopped

1 cup fennel bulb, chopped

2 sweet potatoes, chopped

2 cups vegetable stock

1 bay leaf

Pinch of sea salt

1 tablespoon minced fresh basil

If the weather is damp: Sprinkle with cayenne to taste before serving.

If the weather is dry: Add 1 teaspoon lemon juice when you add the basil.

Heat a large soup pot on medium-high and add the oil. When the oil is warm, add the garlic, leek, fennel, and sweet potatoes, and sauté until the vegetables begin to soften, about 4 minutes. Add the stock, bay leaf, and salt and bring the mixture to a boil. Reduce the heat, cover loosely, and simmer until the vegetables are very tender, about 25 minutes. Remove the bay leaf, add the basil, and puree in a food processor or blender. Serve warm.

MAKES 4 SERVINGS; 104 CALORIES PER SERVING; 2 GRAMS OF FAT; 18 PERCENT OF CALORIES FROM FAT.

potato
"a peeling" to your health

While smoothly slicing spuds into ivory disks, a chef from Peru explained that in the mountains of his country, potatoes are called *Acsumama*, meaning Great Snow Mama, or Great Life Mama. On the high slopes, he continued, corn won't grow, so potatoes are the staple food. Often potatoes are combined in a slowly simmered stew with such grains as quinoa, and flavored with a hot pepper-garlic mix called *ajo*. As he slipped the potatoes into a pot with those very spices, I began to smell the perfume of a warming winter meal.

The importance of potatoes in Peru has spread to the United States, where the tubers are this country's most frequently eaten vegetable. And when they are not deep-fried or slathered with butter or sour cream, potatoes are a wholesome winter choice, containing 220 calories per large baker; iron for energy; vitamin C to help the body absorb the iron; and B vitamins for good nerve health. What's more, potatoes are a good source of soluble fiber to help regulate blood sugar and blood cholesterol levels. For comparison, one peeled potato contains as much soluble fiber as one-third cup of cooked oat bran.

cool spuds

A woman from Hungary taught me to soothe a puffy under-eye area by lying down and applying grated raw potato to the area for 10 minutes. The technique also works to cool topical burns and rashes.

quick cooking tips for potatoes

Top a split and steaming baked potato with fresh salsa. Toss chunks of steamed (for about twelve minutes, or until tender) potato with minced fresh tarragon, minced purple onion, and prepared mustard. Thicken soups by adding one cup of mashed potatoes to every two cups of liquid in the recipe.

potato salad with lentils and fresh mint

In Egypt, mint is often used with beans to increase their digestibility. In addition, the herb adds a reviving taste and aroma to the earthy potato.

If the weather is damp: Increase the garlic to 2 cloves.

3 cups cooked lentils
1 cup cooked cubed potatoes
1 clove garlic, minced
¼ cup minced purple onion
½ cup plain nonfat yogurt or soy
  yogurt

2 teaspoons prepared mustard
Pinch of sea salt
2 tablespoons minced fresh mint

If the weather is dry: Serve on curly red lettuce leaves.

In a medium bowl, combine the lentils, potatoes, garlic, and onion. In a small bowl, stir together the yogurt, mustard, salt, and mint. Pour over the lentil mixture and toss well to combine. Serve warm or at room temperature as a side dish for lunch or dinner.

MAKES 4 SERVINGS; 244 CALORIES PER SERVING; .75 GRAM OF FAT; 4 PERCENT OF CALORIES FROM FAT.

roasted potato salad with capers and chives

If the weather is damp: Add a splash of hot pepper sauce when whisking the lemon juice mixture.

If the weather is dry: Stir in chopped fresh or canned tomato when combining the lemon juice mixture with the potatoes.

Potatoes are a good source of potassium, but boiling can deplete more than half of their nutrient content. The alternative is steaming, thus preserving the potassium, which is said to help prevent high blood pressure, stroke, and heart disease.

1 pound potatoes, cut into chunks and steamed

2 teaspoons olive oil

2 teaspoons capers, drained and minced

1 clove garlic, minced

2 tablespoons minced fresh chives

Juice of 1 lemon

1 teaspoon prepared mustard

Pinch of sea salt

Preheat the broiler. Then, in a bowl, toss the potatoes with the olive oil and spread them out on a cookie sheet and broil, turning frequently, until mottled with brown, about 12 minutes.

In a medium bowl, combine the potatoes, capers, garlic, and chives. In a small bowl, whisk together the lemon, mustard, and salt and toss with the potatoes. Serve warm as a side dish for lunch or dinner.

MAKES 4 SERVINGS; 150 CALORIES PER SERVING; 2.25 GRAMS OF FAT; 15 PERCENT OF CALORIES FROM FAT.

oven fries

Potatoes are a dense and hearty winter food that needs little oil to be satisfying. Here's a quick substitute for the popular but fatty French fries.

4 medium potatoes, sliced into
spears
3 tablespoons skim or soy milk

Pinch of sea salt
Freshly ground black pepper to taste
Malt vinegar for serving

Preheat the oven to 425°F.

In a bowl, toss the spears with the milk, salt, and pepper, and arrange them on a lightly oiled cookie sheet. Bake until tender, about 45 minutes. Serve warm, sprinkled with the vinegar, as a side dish for lunch or dinner.

MAKES 4 SERVINGS; 230 CALORIES PER SERVING; NO ADDED FAT.

If the weather is damp: Add a dash of cayenne when tossing the milk with the potatoes.

If the weather is dry: Serve a crisp green salad with the meal.

potato soup with mushrooms and ginger

The deep flavors of mushroom, garlic, bay, and gingerroot make this soup a welcome tonic for a frosty day.

1 quart vegetable stock
1 onion, minced
1 leek, minced
2 carrots, minced
2 potatoes, minced
3 cloves garlic, mashed though a
press

1 celery stalk, including leaves,
minced
1 cup fresh mushrooms, sliced
1 bay leaf
4 slices fresh gingerroot
Pinch of sea salt
1 teaspoon toasted (dark) sesame oil

In a large stockpot, combine all of the ingredients except the oil and bring to a boil. Reduce the heat, cover loosely, and simmer until all of the vegetables are tender, about 30 minutes. Discard the gingerroot, swirl in the sesame oil, and serve warm as a side dish for lunch or dinner.

MAKES 4 SERVINGS; 180 CALORIES PER SERVING; 1 GRAM OF FAT; 5 PERCENT OF CALORIES FROM FAT.

If the weather is damp: Substitute hot chili oil for the sesame oil.

If the weather is dry: Garnish the soup with minced fresh mint.

potato cakes with leeks

If the weather is damp:
Add a clove of minced
garlic when mashing.

———

If the weather is dry:
Serve with a salad of crisp
greens.

Leeks and potatoes combine to create a bold and warming taste. The mustard, which flavors the cakes, provides nerve-calming magnesium.

2 medium potatoes, peeled, chopped, and boiled

2 carrots, chopped and steamed

2 leeks, topped, tailed, and steamed

2 egg whites

2 tablespoons minced fresh parsley

2 teaspoons prepared mustard

Pinch of sea salt

In a medium bowl, mash together the potatoes, carrots, and leeks. Add the egg whites, parsley, mustard, and salt as you go.

Wet your hands and use the mixture to form firm cakes, about the size of burgers.

Meanwhile, heat a well-seasoned cast-iron pan on medium heat. If you don't have a cast-iron pan, use whatever pan you've got, lightly oiled. Set the cakes in the pan and sizzle until cooked through, about 3 minutes on each side. Serve warm as a side dish for lunch or dinner. Or serve for breakfast or brunch drizzled with plain nonfat yogurt.

MAKES 4 SERVINGS; 125 CALORIES PER SERVING; 1/2 GRAM OF FAT; 6 PERCENT OF CALORIES FROM FAT.

chick-pea and potato curry

Indian spice combinations, or curries, help warm the body by increasing circulation. In addition, curries are useful for "opening" a stuffy winter head. When buying curry powder, smell it first. It should be rich, aromatic, and spicy. If it's not, it's stale and you should seek another brand.

1 pound potatoes, cubed

1 small onion, sliced

2 cloves garlic, minced

½ cup chopped collards, kale, or other hearty greens

1 cup cooked or canned chick-peas (drained)

1 tablespoon canola oil

1 teaspoon good-quality curry powder

Pinch of freshly grated nutmeg

1 tablespoon lemon juice

2 tablespoons tomato sauce

1 tablespoon skim, whole, or soy milk

Pinch of sea salt

If the weather is damp: Add cayenne to taste when sautéing the spice mixture.

If the weather is dry: Sprinkle with minced fresh cilantro before serving.

Steam the potatoes, onion, garlic, collards, and chick-peas over boiling water until the potatoes are tender, about 10 minutes.

Meanwhile, preheat a sauté pan on medium-high and add the oil. When the oil is warm, add the curry powder, nutmeg, lemon juice, and tomato sauce and whisk constantly until they're fragrant and heated through, about 2 minutes. Pour over the potato mixture, add the milk and salt, and toss well to combine. Serve warm as a lunch or dinner entrée.

MAKES 4 SERVINGS; 175 CALORIES PER SERVING; 4 GRAMS OF FAT; 20 PERCENT OF CALORIES FROM FAT.

bread
kneaded for good health

In many remote parts of the globe, I have relied on bread and water for sustenance. Often thought of as plain fare, bread has kept this vegetarian happily satisfied when the only alternative was very old (and I don't mean aged) meat. In the chill of the night I have dined on unleavened whole wheat disks in the Egyptian desert; eaten steamed rice bread for breakfast on a frosty Taipei morning; packed corn bread for my meals while open-boating in the drizzly islands around Honduras.

But I am not the first hungry soul to rely on bread. In Hebrew myth, eating bread is said to bring a divine life, and even salvation. With fish and wine, bread made up the sacramental meal. In ancient Greece, the first loaf of bread from the newly harvested wheat was dedicated to Demeter, an earth deity, to ensure the success of future crops. Some Italian children are advised to kiss bread that they accidentally have dropped upon the floor, lest they be considered wasteful.

Perhaps bread has been a popular staple for thousands of years because people feel good when they eat it. Loaves made of whole grains, such as whole wheat, are a good source of nerve-soothing B vitamins. In addition, eating slices from these wholesome, hearty loaves helps the brain release the hormone serotonin, which makes us feel balanced and in a pleasant mood.

not by bread alone

I am charmed by an activity some school districts call the "edible school yard," where children learn to plant and raise vegetables. For the harvest party the children gather their crops and make a meal for themselves and invited friends, for which each child learns to bake bread. The focus is on the ritual and service of preparing and sharing food. It is also thought by proponents of this program that if a child learns to bake bread, he or she will never be hungry.

quick cooking tips for bread

Try the following loaves for morning toast; sliced, wrapped, and carried to work for healthful snacks; sliced for sandwiches; or made into garlic bread to accompany a warming winter soup.

one-hour two-grain bread

If the weather is damp:
Toast slices and spread
with roasted garlic for an
evening snack.

If the weather is dry:
Spread with all-fruit apple
butter for breakfast or a
snack.

The preparation of this loaf is stress-free, and it has a pleasing crunchy texture and nutty taste. The recipe is based on formulas for Irish soda bread, and it is yeast-free.

½ cup whole wheat bread flour

¾ cup unbleached white flour

⅓ cup yellow cornmeal

¼ cup wheat germ

¼ cup wheat bran

1¼ teaspoons baking soda

½ teaspoon sea salt

1 cup buttermilk, skim, or soy milk

2 tablespoons pure maple syrup

1 egg, beaten; or 2 egg whites

Preheat the oven to 375°F. Lightly oil an 8 × 4-inch loaf pan.

In a large bowl, combine all the dry ingredients. Stir well to combine.

In a small bowl, combine the buttermilk, maple syrup, and egg and mix well. Pour the buttermilk mixture into the flour mixture and use a large rubber spatula to combine well; about 20 strokes should do.

Scoop the batter into the prepared pan, level it off, and bake until the bread is lightly browned and the bottom sounds hollow when you thump it with your finger, about 35 minutes. For a crunchier crust, remove the loaf from the pan and set it directly on the oven rack to bake for the last 10 minutes. Let the bread cool before slicing. (This bread tastes great toasted and spread with hummus for a snack.)

MAKES 1 LOAF, OR 10 SLICES; 90 CALORIES PER SLICE; LESS THAN 1 GRAM OF FAT; 9 PERCENT OF CALORIES FROM FAT.

easy italian-style bread

Half of the flour in these loaves is whole wheat—making it a tonic for digestion and a supplier of calming B vitamins.

2 tablespoons yeast	2 cups unbleached flour
1 teaspoon honey	2 cups whole wheat flour
1 teaspoon olive oil	½ teaspoon sea salt
2 cups warm water (about 110°F.)	

Pour the yeast into a large bowl and add the honey, olive oil, and ½ cup of the water. Stir until the ingredients dissolve, then add the rest of the water, the flours, and salt, and keep stirring until the mixture becomes a dough.

Tip the dough out onto a lightly floured board and knead until the dough becomes satiny, about 10 minutes, adding more flour if necessary. Shape the dough into a ball and set it in a lightly oiled bowl, turning it so all sides have touched the oil. Cover with plastic wrap and let the dough rise in a warm, draft-free place for about an hour.

Preheat the oven to 400°F. Lightly oil a cookie sheet.

Halve the dough and roll out each half on a floured surface to a 12 × 7-inch rectangle. Roll each rectangle, jelly-roll style, into a long baguette and set it seam side down on the prepared cookie sheet. Slice about nine ¼-inch diagonal slits in each loaf, then mist each with water from a spray bottle. This will help make crustier loaves. Bake until lightly browned, for about 40 minutes, misting again after the first 20 minutes. Let the loaves cool before slicing. Sliced thick or thin, this loaf makes great garlic bread. Enjoy it for an indoor winter picnic with a side dish of garlicky beans and a hearty vegetable soup.

MAKES 2 LOAVES, OR 20 SLICES; 90 CALORIES PER SLICE; 2 GRAMS OF FAT; 20 PERCENT OF CALORIES FROM FAT.

If the weather is damp: Toast some slices and spread with a spicy spread, such as Kung Fu Tofu (page 211, Summer).

If the weather is dry: Serve some slices with chopped fresh or canned tomato and basil.

glazed whole wheat challah

If the weather is damp: Enjoy the challah with spicy cinnamon tea.

If the weather is dry: Use the challah to make French toast.

Preparing and baking this high-fiber version of the traditional loaf is what some people call winter therapy. As the bread is kneaded and braided, and hands work the warm, moist dough, you may be able to release unwanted stress.

1 package rapid rise yeast

About 3½ cups unbleached flour

About 3½ cups whole wheat bread flour

1 teaspoon sea salt

1½ cups warm water (about 110°F.)

⅓ cup canola oil

1 tablespoon honey

3 eggs, beaten; or 6 egg whites

1 egg white beaten with a splash of water, for the glaze

In a large bowl, combine the yeast, 3 cups of each flour (6 cups total), and the salt. Then pour in the water, oil, honey, and eggs, and combine well.

Tip the dough out onto a lightly floured surface and knead for about 6 minutes, gradually kneading in extra flour if the dough is too sticky to work. The dough should be smooth and a bit stiff, for easy braiding.

Set the dough into a lightly oiled bowl and roll it over so all the sides have touched the oil. Cover with plastic wrap and let rise until the dough has doubled in size, 30 to 40 minutes.

Punch down the dough and slice it in half. Then slice each half into thirds. Roll each third into a 14-inch-long log. It's easy to do this with floured hands on a lightly floured counter. Braid together 3 logs, pinching the ends closed. Do the same for the remaining 3 logs. Set both braided loaves on a large cookie sheet that has been lined with parchment paper. Let rise uncovered until doubled in size, 30 to 40 minutes.

Meanwhile, preheat the oven to 350°F.

When the loaves are ready, brush them with the glaze. You may not need it all. Bake until the loaves are burnished, 45 to 50 minutes. Let them cool on a wire rack before slicing and serving as is, as a sandwich bread, as toast, or as French toast.

MAKES 2 LOAVES, OR ABOUT 24 SLICES; (WITH WHOLE EGGS) 161 CALORIES PER SLICE; 4.7 GRAMS OF FAT; 26 PERCENT OF CALORIES FROM FAT.

french-style baguettes

The combination of whole wheat and unbleached flours gives these loaves a hearty, high-fiber nutritional profile, without being overly heavy.

2 tablespoons yeast

2 teaspoons honey

2 tablespoons olive oil

1 cup warm water (110°F.)

1 cup warm skim milk or soy milk

About 2½ cups whole wheat bread flour

About 2½ cups unbleached flour

1 teaspoon sea salt

1 egg white

1 teaspoon water

If the weather is damp: Add 2 cloves of minced garlic to the glaze.

If the weather is dry: Serve some slices with a small dish of herbed olive oil for dipping.

In a large bowl, combine the yeast, honey, olive oil, ½ cup each of the water and milk, and about 2 tablespoons of flour. Whisk until the yeast has dissolved, then cover with plastic wrap until bubbly, 10 to 15 minutes.

Whisk in the rest of the water and milk, then gradually add the rest of the flour with the salt. When the whisk becomes gummy, switch to a large rubber spatula and continue to combine the flour with the liquids.

To knead, flour your hands and a counter and turn the dough out onto it. Knead for about 8 minutes, adding more flour if and when necessary. Set the dough into a large oiled bowl and turn it so all sides have touched the oil. Cover with plastic wrap and let rise until the dough has doubled in size, about 30 minutes.

Divide the dough in half, roll each half into a 12 × 6-inch rectangle, and roll up. Set seam side down into 2 lightly oiled French baguette pans. If you don't have baguette pans, set the bread on an oiled cookie sheet, but the finished shapes will be less dramatic. Cover with a tent of plastic wrap that's been propped up with glasses around the outside edges, and let the loaves rise until they double in size, about 30 minutes. Meanwhile, preheat the oven to 450°F. Combine the egg white and the teaspoon of water in a small bowl.

Use a pastry brush to paint the baguettes with the egg white wash; then bake the bread for 15 minutes. Lower the temperature to 350°F. and bake until the baguettes are golden and cooked through, about 30 additional minutes. Let them cool before slicing. Serve with a hearty winter soup; or make into croutons.

MAKES 2 LOAVES, OR 24 SLICES; 103 CALORIES PER SLICE; 1.5 GRAMS OF FAT; 13 PERCENT OF CALORIES FROM FAT.

glazed whole wheat raisin bread

The wheat and raisins in this recipe combine to make a high-fiber bread that helps avert winter constipation.

If the weather is damp: Add I teaspoon ground cinnamon to the dough before kneading, or toast some slices for breakfast or a snack.

If the weather is dry: Use some slices to make French toast, then top with fresh orange sections before serving.

½ cup medium cracked wheat

1½ cups hot orange juice or water

3 tablespoons canola oil

2 tablespoons pure maple syrup

1 tablespoon yeast

¼ cup wheat germ

2 cups whole wheat flour

2 cups unbleached flour

1 teaspoon sea salt

¼ cup raisins

1 tablespoon skim milk for the glaze

In a large bowl, combine the cracked wheat, orange juice or water, and canola oil and let the mixture stand until the wheat has absorbed most of the liquid, about 10 minutes. Stir in the maple syrup and yeast, cover with plastic wrap, and let stand for about 10 minutes. Stir in the wheat germ, flours, and salt until well combined. Then let the dough rest for about 5 minutes so the grains can absorb more liquid.

Flour your hands and a counter and turn the dough out onto it. Knead for about 10 minutes, adding more flour if necessary and kneading in the raisins midway. Set the dough in an oiled bowl and turn the dough around so all sides are coated. Cover with plastic wrap and let the dough rise until it has doubled in size, about 50 minutes.

Punch down the dough and set it into an oiled 9 × 5-inch loaf pan. Cover with a plastic wrap tent that's propped up with glasses around the edges and let the dough rise for about 30 minutes more.

Meanwhile, preheat the oven to 350°F.

Use a pastry brush to paint the top of the loaf with the milk, then bake until the bottom of the loaf sounds hollow when you thump it with your finger, about 55 minutes. Let it cool before slicing. Great for morning toast, or pack 2 slices and take to work for a nourishing midmorning or midafternoon snack.

MAKES 1 LOAF, OR 12 SLICES; 234 CALORIES PER SLICE; 5 GRAMS OF FAT; 20 PERCENT OF CALORIES FROM FAT.

millet biscuits with rosemary

In England in the 1600s, rosemary was prescribed by doctors to those with "cold diseases and giddiness." Modern science knows rosemary is a tonic to "warm" digestion, and those who cook with this herb know that its aroma may be warming to the heart.

1 cup whole wheat flour
1½ cups unbleached flour
1 teaspoon baking soda
½ teaspoon sea salt
1 teaspoon cream of tartar
2 teaspoons minced fresh rosemary,
　or 1 teaspoon dried

1 cup cooked millet
2 tablespoons canola oil
2 egg whites
½ cup plain nonfat yogurt or soy
　yogurt

If the weather is damp: Add 2 cloves of minced garlic to the dough.

If the weather is dry: Serve the biscuits with a creamy spread, such as White Bean Spread with Basil (page 264, Autumn).

Preheat the oven to 425°F. Lightly oil a baking sheet.

In a large bowl, combine the flours, baking soda, salt, cream of tartar, rosemary, and millet. In a medium bowl, whisk together the oil, egg whites, and yogurt. Add the wet ingredients to the dry and use your hands to knead the dough just until it's smooth.

Lightly flour a countertop and, using a floured rolling pin, roll the dough out to a ¼-inch thickness. Cut it into 2½-inch rounds. Set the rounds on the prepared baking sheet and bake them until they're puffed and slightly golden, about 15 minutes. Let the biscuits cool on a wire rack before serving. Great for snacks, or with warming winter soups.

MAKES ABOUT 30 BISCUITS; 60 CALORIES PER BISCUIT; 1 GRAM OF FAT; 15 PERCENT OF CALORIES FROM FAT.

buttermilk corn bread

If the weather is damp: Top the warm wedges with spicy tomato salsa.

If the weather is dry: Serve fresh orange segments for dessert.

Although corn is a cooling, summer crop, when it is ground into flour and baked, it becomes a warming and nourishing winter food.

½ cup unbleached flour

½ cup whole wheat flour

1 cup yellow cornmeal

2 teaspoons baking powder

½ teaspoon baking soda

¼ teaspoon sea salt

1¼ cups buttermilk, skim milk, or
  soy milk

2 egg whites

1 tablespoon canola oil

2 tablespoons pure maple syrup

1 onion, finely chopped

Preheat the oven to 425°F. Lightly oil a 9-inch glass pie pan.

In a large bowl, combine the dry ingredients, stirring to mix well. In a medium bowl, combine the buttermilk, egg whites, oil, maple syrup, and onion and stir well.

Scoop the batter into the prepared pan, smoothing the top with a spatula. Bake until the top is golden and a knife comes out clean when inserted, 20 to 25 minutes. Let the bread cool in the pan on a wire rack for about 5 minutes before slicing into wedges and serving. Enjoy for brunch, or with soup for lunch or dinner.

MAKES 8 SERVINGS; 150 CALORIES PER SERVING; 3 GRAMS OF FAT; 18 PERCENT OF CALORIES FROM FAT.

spicy corn muffins

These little snacks are a warming winter tonic, thanks to the garlic and jalapeños they contain.

1 cup yellow cornmeal

1 cup unbleached flour

1 tablespoon baking powder

½ teaspoon sea salt

2 egg whites

1 cup buttermilk, skim milk, or soy milk

2 tablespoons honey

2 cloves garlic, mashed through a
   press

1 or 2 jalapeño peppers, seeded and
   minced

If the weather is damp: Serve the muffins warm with spicy orange tea.

If the weather is dry: Serve the muffins with a crisp green salad.

Preheat the oven to 375°F. Lightly oil a 12-cup muffin tin.

In a large bowl, combine the dry ingredients and stir well. In a medium bowl, whisk together the egg whites, buttermilk, honey, garlic, and jalapeños. Add the wet ingredients to the dry, using a large rubber spatula to combine them well.

Scoop the batter into the muffin tins and bake until the muffins are lightly browned and cooked through, 20 to 25 minutes. Let the muffins rest in the pan for about 5 minutes, then remove them to a wire rack to finish cooling. Enjoy with brunch, lunch, or dinner. Or pack a muffin and take it to work for a reviving midafternoon snack.

MAKES 12 MUFFINS; 80 CALORIES PER MUFFIN; .75 GRAM OF FAT; 10 PERCENT OF CALORIES FROM FAT.

baked garlic bread

If the weather is damp: Add freshly ground pepper to taste when you add the salt.

If the weather is dry: Add a tablespoon of minced fresh parsley when you add the salt.

This bread can be prepared and baked in about 1 hour, all the while perfuming the house with warming aromas.

1 cup unbleached flour

1 cup whole wheat flour

1 tablespoon baking powder

½ teaspoon sea salt

5 cloves garlic, minced

⅓ cup grated nonfat mozzarella or nonfat soy cheese

1 tablespoon olive oil

2 egg whites

¾ cup buttermilk, skim milk, or soy milk

Preheat the oven to 375°F. Lightly oil an 8½-inch round cake pan.

In a large bowl, stir together the flours, baking powder, sea salt, garlic, and cheese. In a medium bowl, combine the oil, egg whites, and buttermilk. Add the wet ingredients to the dry and mix, using a large rubber spatula. When the dough becomes too stiff, use your hands and continue to mix, forming the dough into a ball.

Press the dough into the prepared pan using a sharp knife to make 8 wedge-shaped cuts about ¼ inch deep. Bake until the bread is light brown, 35 to 40 minutes. Remove the bread from the pan and let it cool on a wire rack before slicing into wedges. Serve warm with stews and soups for lunch or dinner. Or split a warmed wedge and top with grilled winter vegetables for a lunch or dinner entrée.

MAKES 8 SERVINGS; 141 CALORIES PER SERVING; 2 GRAMS OF FAT; 13 PERCENT OF CALORIES FROM FAT.

buckwheat
the warming grain

An herbalist from Korea was stirring a vat of buckwheat cream—one cup of buckwheat groats simmered in ten cups of water for one hour—while she explained that very ill people—cancer patients, for instance—often develop malnutrition because their digestive system is "cold" and they can't absorb nutrients. The buckwheat cream, she said, provides a solution, offering an easily digestible source of nourishment, including magnesium for nerve health and stable blood pressure; potassium for alertness and stable blood sugar levels; and vitamin E to help strengthen the heart and skin. One serving of buckwheat, about half a cup cooked, contains 91 calories and only a trace of fat. In addition, buckwheat has a warming, energizing effect on the entire body, making this grain a great winter food choice for anyone.

but what is it?

Buckwheat is not a wheat; in fact, it is not even truly a grain. Buckwheat is a seed, originating in Asia and spreading thence to Russia and Poland.

✤ ***quick cooking tips for buckwheat***

This grain's rich and nutty taste can be used instead of rice in side dishes, soups, stews, casseroles, and stir fries. Buckwheat flour is famous as the main ingredient in Japanese soba noodles, and it is also delicious when used (half and half with unbleached white flour) in recipes for pancakes, waffles, and crepes. To cook buckwheat, toast one cup of groats in a large, dry cast-iron or nonstick pan on high heat, until they're fragrant and lightly browned. Carefully add two cups of water or vegetable stock and bring to a boil. Reduce the heat and cover loosely. Let the buckwheat simmer until tender, about fifteen minutes. You'll have about two and half cups of cooked buckwheat.

vanilla-scented buckwheat pancakes

If the weather is damp: Add I teaspoon ground cinnamon to the batter.

If the weather is dry: Serve with sliced ripe pears.

Breakfasting on these pancakes can energize you on even the dullest wintry day, since they are a good source of B vitamins, which help the body produce uplifting adrenaline.

3/4 **cup unbleached flour**
3/4 **cup whole wheat pastry flour**
Pinch of sea salt
1 1/2 **teaspoons baking powder**
1 cup cooked and cooled buckwheat
1 1/2 **cups buttermilk, skim milk, or soy milk**

3 tablespoons honey
3 egg whites
1 tablespoon canola oil
1 teaspoon pure vanilla extract

In a medium bowl, combine the dry ingredients and stir well. In another medium bowl, whisk together the buttermilk, honey, egg whites, oil, and vanilla. Pour the wet ingredients into the dry and stir until just combined. Spray a nonstick pan with nonstick spray and heat on medium high. Make pancakes using 3 tablespoons of batter for each one. Let each cook until bubbles form on top, about 2 minutes, then flip and cook until the second side is lightly browned, 1 1/2 to 2 minutes more. Serve warm for breakfast or brunch.

MAKES 4 SERVINGS; 330 CALORIES PER SERVING; 5 GRAMS OF FAT; 14 PERCENT OF CALORIES FROM FAT.

buckwheat pudding with dark honey

Tinged with the comforting scent of vanilla, this recipe makes a wholesome winter breakfast, snack, or dessert.

2 cups cooked buckwheat

1 cup skim or lowfat soy milk

¼ cup dark honey

1 teaspoon pure vanilla extract

¼ teaspoon lemon zest

Pinch of sea salt

If the weather is damp: Add ½ teaspoon of freshly grated nutmeg before baking.

If the weather is dry: Serve with chilled orange sections.

Preheat the oven to 350°F. Lightly oil a 1-quart baking dish. Combine all of the ingredients in the prepared dish and stir well. Bake until set, about 45 minutes. Serve warm for breakfast or brunch.

MAKES 4 SERVINGS; 108 CALORIES PER SERVING; TRACE OF FAT.

buckwheat pilaf with garlic and leek

This high-fiber dish can help keep an otherwise sluggish winter digestive tract toned and healthy.

1 tablespoon olive oil

2 cloves garlic, minced

2 carrots, diced

1 leek, topped, tailed, and minced

1 cup buckwheat groats

Pinch of sea salt

2½ cups vegetable stock

2 scallions, minced

1 teaspoon balsamic vinegar

If the weather is damp: Stir in a splash of hot pepper sauce with the scallions.

If the weather is dry: During the last 5 minutes of cooking, add ½ cup chopped broccoli.

Heat a medium soup pot on medium-high and add the oil. When the oil is warm, add the garlic, carrots, leek, and buckwheat, and sauté until the ingredients are fragrant and the vegetables are slightly wilted, about 3 minutes. Add the salt and stock, and bring to a boil. Reduce the heat to medium-low and simmer, loosely covered, until the buckwheat is tender and the liquid has been absorbed, about 45 minutes. Stir in the scallions and vinegar and serve warm as a side dish for lunch or dinner.

MAKES 4 SERVINGS; 155 CALORIES PER SERVING; 3.5 GRAMS OF FAT; 20 PERCENT OF CALORIES FROM FAT.

soba noodles with spicy peanut sauce

Soba are Japanese noodles made with buckwheat flour. They are a good winter fortifier, containing nerve-soothing B vitamins and calcium.

If the weather is damp: Sprinkle the soba with minced scallions before serving.

If the weather is dry: Sprinkle the soba with minced fresh cilantro before serving.

1 tablespoon peanut butter
1 tablespoon prepared mustard
1 tablespoon lime juice
1 tablespoon hot pepper sauce
1 clove garlic, minced

1 tablespoon reduced–sodium soy
  sauce
1 tablespoon vegetable stock or
  water
8 ounces soba noodles, cooked

In a medium bowl, whisk together all the ingredients except the noodles. Toss the sauce with the noodles and serve warm as a lunch or dinner entrée.

MAKES 4 SERVINGS; 331 CALORIES PER SERVING; 2 GRAMS OF FAT; 6 PERCENT OF CALORIES FROM FAT.

citrus
antidote for dryness

My Chinese and Ayurvedic teachers continually tease me about eating citrus in winter. "Citrus is cooling," they criticize, and question why I eat it in cold weather. The simple reason is that citrus is hydrating, and in the dry, artificial heat of indoor homes and offices, fresh orange sections and moist tangerines are, for me, a rejuvenating snack. I bring citrus along on winter train trips to New York; stock up on citrus for automobile journeys; and pack citrus in plastic bags for a refreshment on plane trips. For people who wake on a winter morning with dry eyes, parched skin, and scratchy throat, eating a cool, fresh orange is an instant remedy.

Japanese legend seems in tune with my point of view on citrus, regarding the orange as a symbol for the ever-golden, health-giving sun, and a provider of good fortune and immortality. For a modern take on the orange's attributes: One fruit contains a mere 62 calories and virtually no fat. It's a good source of immune-enhancing vitamin C, digestion-toning fiber, and body-strengthening folate. Eating a sweet, juicy orange for dessert is a satisfying, low-fat choice that can aid in weight loss and (due to the vitamin C) boost your absorption of plant-based iron by 400 percent.

make a wish

The orange blossom is the January 26 birthday flower, symbolizing purity, worthiness, and eternal love.

quick cooking tips for oranges

Stir the fresh sections from a whole orange into one serving of cooked morning oatmeal. Add the sections from two whole oranges to a green salad to serve four; heat orange juice instead of water for making tea.

revitalizing citrus salad

If the weather is damp: Add a 2-inch cinnamon stick to the bottom of the bowl before refrigerating.

If the weather is dry: Garnish with fresh mint leaves.

Make this hydrating tonic ahead, to give the fruit juices time to mingle.

2 large navel oranges, peeled and sectioned

2 tangerines, peeled and sectioned

1 cup seedless grapes

Juice of 1 lemon

In a glass dish, mix all of the ingredients and stir to combine. Cover and refrigerate overnight or for at least an hour. Serve the salad slightly chilled with breakfast, or as a dessert for lunch or dinner. If the air in your office is parched and drying, pack a serving to take along for a revitalizing snack.

MAKES 4 SERVINGS; 66 CALORIES PER SERVING; NO ADDED FAT.

refreshing citrus dressing

This uplifting condiment is what aromatherapists call a "euphoric," a substance containing aromas that rejuvenate the mood. Toss with fresh greens or steamed winter vegetables.

If the weather is damp: Add hot pepper sauce to taste.

¼ cup white wine vinegar
¼ cup fresh lemon juice
¼ cup fresh orange juice
1 tablespoon grated lime zest

½ teaspoon prepared mustard
Pinch of sea salt
Freshly ground black pepper

If the weather is dry: Add minced fresh parsley, to taste, before serving.

In a glass jar, combine all of the ingredients, cover, and shake well. Stored refrigerated, the dressing will keep for up to 5 days.

MAKES ¾ CUP, OR SIX 2-TABLESPOON SERVINGS; 6 CALORIES PER SERVING; NO ADDED FAT.

Cooking is a great winter activity. Simmering kettles of aromatic veg-etables, grains, and herbs send warm and nourishing aromas through the house, creating a restful feeling of well-being. These menus will help you start to plan winter meals; then use your instincts to create your own combinations and recipes.

Restful Winter Brunch or Dinner: The carrots and miso in the soup help to soothe stressed digestion. The potatoes offer blood pressure–calming potassium; and the greens offer the mineral magnesium, a natural nerve tonic. This meal makes a good Friday night dinner, especially after a harried week. Set a fancy table, light candles, and invite your sweetheart.

* Carrot-Miso Soup (page 21)
* Potato Cakes with Leeks (page 48)
* Sautéed Beet Greens with Garlic and Ginger (page 36)
* Restful Winter Tea (page 11) or Deep Spirits Tea (page 10)

Immune-Boosting Winter Lunch or Dinner: If you're pressed for time, make the brown rice dish on Sunday, and keep it covered and refrig-erated for up to a week, reheating as needed. It's a good source of folate, a nutrient important to the immune system, and also critical for pregnant women, as folate aids fetal growth. The dish is also a good introduction to vegetarian food for family and friends, because it's tasty and the ingredients are not exotic. As to the accompani-ments, the hot peppers and garlic in the soup, and the mashed parsnips, help ward off colds and flu; and the sweet potatoes are an excellent source of beta carotene, to fight stuffy noses.

* Spicy Sweet Potato Soup (page 41)
* Brown Rice with Fragrant Vegetables (page 18)
* Garlic-Mashed Parsnips (page 25)
* (Romaine with) Refreshing Citrus Dressing (page 67)

Energy-Boosting Winter Lunch: The spices in these recipes contain thermogenic, or heat-producing, compounds that increase circulation and thus give us energy. Make the muffins ahead and freeze them, defrosting as needed to pack for lunch.

* Spicy Corn Muffins (page 59)
* Sweet Potato Soup with Lemongrass and Scallions (page 40)

Nourishing Winter Breakfast: Buckwheat lends a warming and nutritious start to the day, and for those of us parched by indoor heat, the citrus in the salad is a juicy remedy. For convenience, make the pancakes ahead and freeze them, individually wrapped. Defrost at room temperature overnight and reheat in a nonstick sauté pan.

* Vanilla-Scented Buckwheat Pancakes (page 62)
* Revitalizing Citrus Salad (page 66)

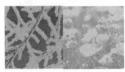

gateway
from winter
to spring

In nature, progress often occurs in small degrees. At thirty-two degrees the earth is frozen and still, but move just one degree higher to thirty-three and the earth starts to warm and thaw. Then plants, whose energies have rested for the winter, begin an ascent that gradually forms new buds. People, too, who have rested their deep roots throughout the winter, now prepare to rise and bloom in spring.

This is a good time to take stock of your health habits and adopt positive new patterns. The ideas in this section will provide that inspiration, and assist you in enjoying the degrees by which winter turns to spring.

Treat Yourself to a Massage—To increase immunities, stimulate circulation, reduce muscle tension and stress, and improve joint mobility after a cold, wet winter, make an appointment with a massage therapist. Ask friends or your doctor for recommendations, or visit local clinics or spas to review the facilities before making an appointment. Look in the phone book for certified massage school listings, and call for recommendations. Make your appointment for later in the day, so you can go home and relax for the evening afterward. In addition, many experts advise eating lightly after a massage—a green salad or fruit salad—and drinking lots of fresh water with lemon slices added to help flush any accumulated toxins from your system.

Take a Walk—To help adapt to the pending warmer weather, and to avoid illness by building immunities, take a walk outside each day for about 20 minutes. Wear a jacket and keep your neck wrapped even if you feel warm. If not, your body will generate too much heat (to keep you warm) and you'll wind up being fatigued from the extra energy output.

Play in Mud—If you have a garden, start working the soil. Turn it; rake in composted cow manure to make it richer; work in sand and peat if you've got too much clay; dig out a space for a new herb garden. Inside, trim and prune your houseplants, feed them, buy them a present of a plant sprayer and mist them daily with fresh water.

Adopt an Herb—Gingerroot contains aromatic properties that help increase circulation, giving the body energy and helping to alleviate aches and pains. Add a quarter teaspoon of ground ginger to a cup of tea or coffee; chew on a piece of candied ginger several times a day; add three fresh gingerroot slices to a glass of room temperature water before drinking. Cayenne has similar properties, and in addition it helps to treat sluggish digestion. Add a pinch to a cup of hot tea into which you've squeezed the juice of half a lemon; take a small bottle of cayenne with you and shake it, to taste, into restaurant soups or atop salads, pasta, and rice dishes. To enhance your immunities, add minced fresh garlic to taste to spreads, dips, salad dressings, and tuna, chicken, egg, and tofu salads; ask for extra garlic when ordering at Chinese, Thai, Vietnamese, and Italian restaurants. To help fight stress, begin to use more mustard in your cooking. It is a very good source of the mineral magnesium, whose absence in the diet is associated with seasonal irritability, anxiety, and depression. Add a tablespoon of prepared mustard to a quarter cup of creamy dip or salad dressing; use prepared mustard to coat fish before grilling; fill your pepper mill with half mustard seeds and half peppercorns and grind on salads and into soups and stews.

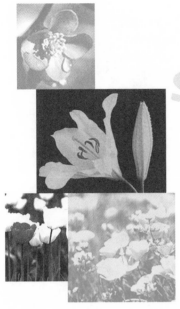

spring:
the season of
renewal

february, march, april

BEST TIME OF YEAR FOR:

❋ *Getting rid of that which you no longer need*

❋ *Creating new ideas*

❋ *Making plans*

In half-light, gliding along the banks of the Wissahickon creek in Pennsylvania one bracing February dawn, I listened as an expert bird watcher explained why spring begins in our second calendar month.

Birds begin to migrate to their northern homes around Valentine's Day, he noted, because the days are getting longer and warmer. Small mammals—squirrels, bunnies, groundhogs—have emerged from their winter nests to stretch in the sun and snack on green shoots. The world is awakening from winter slumber. In fact, on many French, German, and English gardening calendars, February marks the first spring month. And despite the fact that the vernal equinox—when the sun passes over the equator, celestially marking the first day of spring—does not occur until March, the earth knows it's now spring.

People, too, begin to stir with inspiration and energy. After a long winter it's instinctive to be filled with enthusiasm and to freshen, fluff, and clean; activities that behaviorists, following the animals' lead, interestingly call "nesting." A man at my local hardware store confirms this phenomenon, saying that he loves spring because people buy thousands of dollars of cleanup supplies. In addition, travel agents say that spring is the busiest time, with exciting plans afoot for summer journeys. Also engrossed are caterers, hired to arrange upcoming weddings and celebrations.

Spring typifies awakening—it is the "early morning" of the year.

THE MONTH OF FEBRUARY
The name of the second month in our calendar year comes from the Latin *februs*, meaning "to make libations." The custom of February celebrations began with the ancient Romans, who honored the warmth of spring with good cheer and feasts.

INTERESTING DATES IN FEBRUARY
Chinese New Year (date floats) when, during this festival of fire, the light of spring is celebrated with candles and firecrackers.

Imagine this: In Italy, one icon of spring is a young man dressed in black on one side and white on the other, suggesting that spring is light emerging from darkness. He wears a cummerbund of stars and holds a staff entwined with spring herbs and flowers. In Chinese lore and literature, spring is depicted as a turquoise dragon, a silhouette of rolling hills alive with the power of millions of blue-green sprouts.

This spring theory—that as the earth renews itself, so do all its inhabitants—may not prove true for everyone. A winter rich with fatty foods, lack of exercise, overindulgence of alcohol, unmanaged stress, certain medications, or just a bad mood may leave one feeling less than inspired, no matter how fresh the weather. In that case, the suggestions in this chapter may provide encouragement.

first aid kit for spring

To shake off the slower pace of winter, think "new." Try a surprising but flattering new hairstyle, lipstick, or tie. Choose a new attitude. You may also wish to adopt one or more of these reviving tips.

Renew Your Space—Find time to clean out some clutter in your life. Start with one thing—straighten out a kitchen drawer while you're talking on the phone; go through your closet and get rid of any piece of clothing you haven't worn in a year; sort through the "I'll get to this eventually" pile of papers on your desk; reevaluate your association with people who annoy you. Even if you unclutter just one thing in your life, you'll feel, at least temporarily, renewed.

Renew Your Herbal Pantry—Open every dried herb and spice jar you own and smell it. If the aroma is not vibrant and aromatic, compost those old leaves and replace them. Investigate and find new herbs you like, and avoid buying those you've purchased in the past but haven't used. Try peppermint, which has a reviving effect on the body, by adding a teaspoon of dried leaves (or two teaspoons of minced fresh leaves) to a vinaigrette to serve four. Or buy fresh spring herbs, such as borage and burnet, and add the leaves to green salads to taste.

Renew Your Skin—Buy a loofah, or other gentle body scrubber, to help buff dry winter skin away. Use it in the shower with a reviving lemon- or citrus-scented soap, rubbing feet, elbows, knees, and other body parts with soft, circular motions. Be very gentle with facial and neck skin, as a loofah may be too harsh. Instead, rub on your face and neck two tablespoons of thick, plain yogurt, and let it soak in while you're showering. Yogurt contains natural exfoliation properties that won't abrade the skin's surface. Leave it on for up to fifteen minutes, then wash as usual. As for moisturizing, if your skin gets oilier as the weather gets warmer, use half of your usual moisturizer combined with an equal amount of aloe gel. This works for both the face and body, providing hydration without greasiness. Be sure to buy aloe gel, in a bottle or tube, that is free from harsh menthol or artificial colors and fragrances, all of which can irritate facial skin.

Renew Your Body—Is your body bored by its exercise routine? Try something new. If you do mostly aerobic activity, add some stretching. If you do yoga or tai chi, add a brisk walk or an aerobic dance class. If you do nothing, park your car a block farther away from your destination than you usually do and walk the rest of the way; get off the subway several blocks before your stop; walk up a flight of stairs; in the shower, flex your calves by standing first on tiptoe, then on your heels, and repeating ten times (don't slip).

Renew Your Mind—A Pima Indian I met in Sedona, Arizona, told me that "the world rearranges itself to accommodate your picture of reality." What he meant was, it's all attitude—how *you* see the events in your life determines whether you're going to be in a good mood or in a bad mood. Then, no matter what happens, you can choose how you feel. When a stressful situation occurs, you might choose to feel calm, free, and optimistic rather than tight, controlled, and tense.

INTERESTING DATES IN APRIL

April 1—*All Fools' Day,* an ancient agrarian feast celebrating awakening and rejuvenation, noted for humorous pranks and fun. *April 15*—*St. Ruadan's Day,* an ancient Celtic holiday where it was believed that wild birds celebrated because their "fetters were at last unlocked" from winter's cold prison. *April 20* (approximate)—The sun enters the zodiac sign of Taurus, the celestial bull, symbolizing growth and fertility. *April 30*—Ancient Celts remained awake all night to welcome the festival of *Beltane,* which begins at dawn on May 1.

INTERESTING DATES IN MARCH

March 5—*Festival of Kites* in China and Japan, where people fly dragon or fish kites to symbolize strength and longevity with the winds of spring. *March 21*—*The vernal equinox,* when night and day are the same length. On this day the sun moves into the zodiac sign of Aries, the heavenly ram, symbolizing the birth of new ideas and thoughts. *March 27*—*Smell the Wind Day* in Egypt, where upon rising in the morning, participants immediately smell a spring onion, which is thought to promote good health. Later they picnic outdoors, enjoying fresh spring breezes.

THE MONTH OF APRIL

The fourth month in our calendar year is from the Latin *aperio,* "to open," because it is the month when the earth opens to produce new gifts.

cleansing spring beverages

"You need a spring tonic," decreed a friend in Rome, as I entered her apartment feeling light-headed and without appetite. She charged immediately to the kitchen where, with a flourish, she peeled a whole lemon in one long swoop, and tossed the peel into a small saucepan with about a cup and a half of water.

Lecturing nonstop, my friend instructed me, for future reference, to boil the tonic until the water was reduced to one cup, about ten minutes, then drink it hot.

"My Portuguese nanny gave this to me for stomachaches as a child. She called it *cha* for 'tea,' the same as the Japanese word," my friend went on. "Spring is the time to nourish the liver, or you wind up feeling like you do. Boiled lemon peel is the best liver tonic—don't they teach you this in Hong Kong? You must come to Italy more often."

Not unlike the Italian and Portuguese, many cultures espouse their own spring tonics to prepare the body and mind for the lighter days of spring. Some interesting versions are offered here.

three-spice tea

East Indian Ayurvedic herbalists recommend this formula to abate such spring digestive woes as bloating, gas, and indigestion.

1 teaspoon cuminseed
1 teaspoon coriander seed

1 teaspoon fennel seed
2 cups water

In a small saucepan, combine all of the ingredients and bring to a boil. Reduce the heat and simmer until the water has been reduced to 1 cup, about 15 minutes. Discard the spices and sip warm, up to 3 times a day.

MAKES ONE SERVING; ABOUT 5 CALORIES PER SERVING; NO ADDED FAT.

If the weather is damp: Stir in a pinch of ground turmeric before sipping.

If the weather is dry: Add a twist of lemon before sipping.

ginger-chive decongestant

In Japan, herbalists recommend this bracing brew to soothe the symptoms of spring allergies and sinus congestion.

4 slices gingerroot
1½ cups water

1 tablespoon minced fresh chives

In a small saucepan, combine the ginger and water and bring to a boil. Continue to boil until the water has been reduced to about 1 cup, about 10 minutes. Remove the pan from the heat, add the chives, cover, and let the brew steep for about 5 minutes. Then discard the ginger and chives and sip warm, up to 3 cups a day.

MAKES ONE SERVING; ABOUT 5 CALORIES PER CUP; NO ADDED FAT.

If the weather is damp: Increase the gingerroot to 6 slices.

If the weather is dry: Use ¾ cup water and ¾ cup orange juice when boiling the gingerroot.

mixed mint tea

If the weather is damp: Add 3 black peppercorns to the tea while steeping.

If the weather is dry: Add a twist of lemon before sipping.

A Jamu herbalist in Indonesia taught me to prepare this spring elixir. The mints and the lemongrass contain aromatic compounds that help soothe spring digestive irritability.

1 teaspoon dried peppermint

1 teaspoon dried spearmint

1 teaspoon dried lemongrass

2 cups hot water

In a teapot, combine all of the ingredients, cover, and steep for 5 minutes. Discard the herbs and sip warm or very slightly chilled, as needed.

MAKES TWO 1-CUP SERVINGS; ABOUT 5 CALORIES PER SERVING; NO ADDED FAT.

tisane of thyme with variations

If the weather is damp: Add a slice of gingerroot while steeping.

If the weather is dry: Add a twist of lemon before sipping.

French herbalists prescribe thyme tea to help rejuvenate the body for spring. The herb's aromatic properties can help prevent coughs, sore throats, colds, and spring flu.

1 teaspoon dried thyme, or
   2 teaspoons fresh

1 cup hot water

Steep the thyme in the water, covered, for 4 minutes. Discard the thyme and sip warm as needed.

MAKES ONE SERVING; ABOUT 3 CALORIES PER SERVING; NO ADDED FAT.

VARIATIONS:

Alleviate spring constipation: Add the juice of ½ lemon before sipping.
Soothe spring aches and pains: Add a pinch of cayenne before sipping.
Calm spring stresses: Add a teaspoon dried chamomile while steeping.
Relieve spring congestion: Add a teaspoon dried peppermint while steeping.

tarragon-mint tonic

The recipe for this refreshing beverage was taught to me by a Kahuna man, or Hawaiian herbalist, on the Big Island of Hawaii. He likes to serve it after dinner to calm digestion, thus promoting peaceful sleep.

1 teaspoon dried tarragon   1 cup hot water
1 teaspoon dried peppermint

Steep the tarragon and mint in the water, covered, for 5 minutes. Discard the plant material, then sip warm or slightly chilled, as needed.

MAKES ONE SERVING; ABOUT 3 CALORIES PER SERVING; NO ADDED FAT.

If the weather is damp: Sip the tonic while it's warm.

If the weather is dry: Add a twist of lemon before sipping.

lemon-parsley "potion" for water retention

English herbalists favor this boiled tea as a natural diuretic to ease bloat and water retention. They caution, however, that the cause of these conditions (salty junk food; lack of adequate water intake) should be addressed.

1 lemon, sliced   3 cups water
½ cup fresh parsley, whole leaves
   and stems

In a small saucepan, combine all of the ingredients and bring to a boil. Continue to boil until the liquid has been reduced to about 2 cups, about 10 minutes. Discard the plant material and sip. You can try up to 3 cups a day.

MAKES TWO 1-CUP SERVINGS; ABOUT 5 CALORIES PER SERVING; NO ADDED FAT.

If the weather is damp: Add a 1-inch cinnamon stick to the pot before boiling, then discard.

If the weather is dry: Sip the "potion" at room temperature or very slightly chilled.

dandelion-mint tonic

If the weather is damp: Stir in a pinch of ground cinnamon before sipping.

If the weather is dry: Add 5 raisins to the tonic before boiling.

This combination is popular with Cherokee herbalists to relieve water retention. Be sure, however, to find out why you're retaining water (review your diet and exercise routine), rather than relying on herbs to cure the condition.

1 tablespoon dried dandelion root   3 cups water
1 teaspoon dried peppermint

In a small saucepan, combine all of the ingredients and bring to a boil. Continue to boil until the liquid has been reduced to 1 cup, about 10 minutes. Discard the plant material and sip. You can have up to 3 cups a day.

MAKES TWO 1-CUP SERVINGS; ABOUT 5 CALORIES PER SERVING; NO ADDED FAT.

soothing catnip tonic

If the weather is damp: Sip the tonic while it's warm.

If the weather is dry: Sip the tonic at room temperature, or very slightly chilled.

A Pennsylvania Dutch woman taught me to pick and dry spring catnip for use as a digestive and upper respiratory tonic. I now take the easy route and buy my catnip, keeping it handy for a quick rejuvenation.

2 teaspoons dried catnip   1 cup hot water

Steep the catnip in the water, covered, for 5 minutes. Discard the catnip and sip warm or slightly chilled, as needed.

MAKES ONE SERVING; ABOUT 3 CALORIES PER CUP; NO ADDED FAT.

ADDITIONS:
To help cool a fever due to spring cough or cold, add 1 teaspoon dried yarrow while steeping.
To calm anxiety, add 1 teaspoon dried chamomile while steeping.
To help break up respiratory congestion, add a pinch of cayenne before sipping.

fresh chervil tonic

This delicately anise-flavored infusion is a popular spring nostrum in Norway, where herbalists say it gently cleans the system. Try it first thing in the morning to start your day refreshed.

2 handfuls (about 1 cup loosely packed) fresh chervil	4 cups water, at room temperature

In a large pitcher, combine the chervil and water and let steep at room temperature overnight. Discard the chervil in the morning, and sip the refreshing brew as desired. Store the tonic, covered and refrigerated, if you're keeping it for more than 1 day.

MAKES FOUR 1-CUP SERVINGS; ABOUT 3 CALORIES PER CUP; NO ADDED FAT.

If the weather is damp: Add a tablespoon of chopped fresh tarragon before steeping.

If the weather is dry: Add 1 slice of lemon before steeping.

roasted barley brew

Japanese and Korean healers recommend this tea to help tonify and cleanse the liver.

3 tablespoons roasted barley (available at Asian markets and natural food stores)	4⅓ cups water

In a medium saucepan, combine the barley and water and bring to a boil. Reduce the heat slightly and continue to simmer until the tea is medium-amber in color, about 10 minutes. Discard the barley and sip warm, at room temperature, or very slightly chilled.

MAKES FOUR 1-CUP SERVINGS; ABOUT 3 CALORIES PER SERVING; NO ADDED FAT.

If the weather is damp: Sip warm with a twist of lemon.

If the weather is dry: Sip slightly chilled, combined with an equal amount of apple juice.

spring stomach soother

If the weather is damp:
Increase the gingerroot to
I teaspoon.

———

If the weather is dry: Add
a lemon twist before
sipping.

I learned this potion from a Japanese herbalist, who explained that the ingredi-ents ease a spring stomachache by neutralizing stomach acids.

¼ teaspoon tamari soy sauce
½ teaspoon umeboshi plum paste
   (available at Asian markets and
   natural food stores)

½ teaspoon finely grated fresh
   gingerroot
1 cup hot water

In a mug, combine all of the ingredients and sip warm.

MAKES ONE SERVING; ABOUT 25 CALORIES PER SERVING; NO ADDED FAT.

cleansing
spring foods

The spring pantry includes fresh herbs and other plants—upward-growing sprouts and shoots—that reflect the rejuvenating energy of the season. Chervil, chives, arugula, mustard greens, cresses, tarragon, mint, and dandelion contain chlorophyll and various aromatics that gently cleanse the body, leaving you free and optimistic to enjoy the freshness of the season. Green beans and peas provide digestion-friendly fiber; and asparagus, radishes, and strawberries contain compounds that gently flush the system, helping to prevent the digestive distress, sinus trouble, and headaches that a winter of eating fried, fatty, and other heavy offerings may have aggravated. To create your own cure, use some or all of these spring offerings to make a cleansing daily salad, dressed with fresh lemon juice, a pinch of sea salt, and a splash of olive oil. Or explore the following suggestions.

spring greens
natural nutrition

In Germany one April, I participated in the "spring cure," a dietary regime where participants sprinkle chopped spring greens on everything they eat—soups, stews, omelets, salads, and sandwiches, just to name a few items. Using dandelion greens, mustard greens, spinach, cresses, chervil, and chives, Germans believe their "spring cure" prevents *Frühjahrsmudigkeit*, or nutrient deficiency resulting from the lack of fresh vegetables and fruits during the winter.

Spring greens are a rich source of beta carotene, vitamin C, chlorophyll, and trace minerals, and adopting them as a seasonal cure is a smart way to help avert digestive distress, headaches, upper respiratory complaints, and complexion problems. Furthermore, half a cup of most spring greens, cooked, contains less than 20 calories, with no added fat.

wild greens

Dandelion, and other spring greens such as chickweed, wild mustard, yarrow, plantain, and wild violet, can all be harvested in the wild. Consult an expert (try your county extension office) to teach you what and where to pick. And be sure to limit harvests to areas that have not been sprayed with pesticides or herbicides.

quick cooking tip for spring greens

To prepare spring greens, boil about an inch of water in a large soup pot, adding about two cups of raw greens for each serving. Cover the pot and steam/boil the greens until they're a bright green and tender; start checking for doneness at one minute. When they're ready, use tongs to remove the greens to a strainer. Then toss with such seasonings as lemon juice and olive oil; or minced sun-dried tomatoes and balsamic vinegar. Eat the greens as a side dish, or toss with hot pasta. Of course, you can also enjoy spring greens raw in salads or sandwiches, or consult the recipes below.

fresh spinach sauce with chives

The spinach in this easy condiment may help avert spring headaches, due to the magnesium it contains. In addition, some herbalists say that the chlorophyll in spinach helps to cleanse the digestive system gently, thus preventing gas, constipation, diarrhea, and spring skin eruptions.

If the weather is damp: Add hot pepper sauce to taste before processing.

If the weather is dry: Add 1 teaspoon lemon juice before processing.

2 cups fresh spinach
2/3 cup buttermilk or plain nonfat
  soy milk

1 tablespoon minced fresh chives
Pinch of sea salt

In a food processor or blender, combine all the ingredients and blend until smooth. Use as a sauce for salmon or other grilled fish; toss with hot pasta; serve atop steamed asparagus.

MAKES 4 SERVINGS; 30 CALORIES PER SERVING; NO ADDED FAT.

udon noodles with spinach ribbons

If the weather is damp:
Add a dried hot pepper to
the stock when simmering.

If the weather is dry:
Sprinkle with minced fresh
chervil before serving.

Udon are Japanese-style whole wheat noodles that are tasty and easy to digest. They contain B vitamins that act as a nerve tonic, helping to banish spring stresses.

8 ounces raw udon noodles
    (available at natural food stores,
    Asian markets, and some
    supermarkets)
1½ cups vegetable stock
2 slices fresh gingerroot

2 cloves garlic, minced
1 teaspoon regular or reduced-
    sodium soy sauce
8 ounces fresh spinach leaves, sliced
    into thin ribbons
5 scallions, minced

Cook the udon by boiling it until just tender, about 4 minutes. Then drain and set aside.

Pour the stock into a large frying pan and add the gingerroot, garlic, and soy sauce. Bring the mixture to a simmer; then add the noodles, spinach, and scallions and heat through, for about 20 seconds. Serve the noodles warm, as a lunch or dinner soup entrée, in shallow bowls with some cooking liquid poured over them.

MAKES 4 SERVINGS; 240 CALORIES PER SERVING; I GRAM OF FAT; 4 PERCENT OF CALORIES FROM FAT.

steamed spinach with spring herbs

Thyme, one of the spring herbs offered here, contains a compound called thy-mol that may help avert some symptoms of spring allergies.

1 pound fresh spinach

1 tablespoon minced fresh thyme,
   or 1½ teaspoons dried

1 tablespoon minced fresh chives

1 carrot, coarsely shredded

1 clove garlic, minced

Pinch of sea salt

Juice of ½ lemon

If the weather is damp: Sprinkle on freshly ground pepper before serving.

If the weather is dry: Serve the spinach very slightly chilled with extra lemon wedges for drizzling.

Steam the spinach over boiling water until the leaves are bright green and just tender. Start checking at about 1½ minutes—young, tender leaves will take less time than older ones.

Tip the spinach into a bowl along with the remaining ingredients, and toss well to combine. Serve warm or at room temperature as a side dish, as an appetizer atop crusty sliced bread, or as a filling for crepes.

MAKES 4 SERVINGS; 26 CALORIES PER SERVING; NO ADDED FAT.

linguine with fresh spinach

If the weather is damp:
Add hot pepper sauce to
taste to the spinach
mixture during sautéing.

If the weather is dry: Serve
with a crisp cucumber
salad.

This recipe has a fresh, springlike look that appeals even to those who don't love greens. The garlic helps banish spring aches and pains by increasing circulation.

2 teaspoons olive oil

3 cloves garlic, minced

2 cups fresh spinach

4 ripe tomatoes, cored and finely chopped

4 cups hot, cooked linguine (about ½ pound uncooked)

2 tablespoons freshly grated Parmesan or soy Parmesan for sprinkling

Heat a sauté pan on medium-high and warm the olive oil. Add the garlic, spinach, and tomatoes and sauté until the vegetables are beginning to wilt, about 3 minutes. Immediately toss with the linguine, sprinkle with the Parmesan, and serve warm for lunch or dinner.

MAKES 4 SERVINGS; 270 CALORIES PER SERVING; 4 GRAMS OF FAT; 15 PERCENT OF CALORIES FROM FAT.

spring greens soup

This tonic-in-a-soup contains watercress, a delicate green that offers insoluble fiber to help prevent spring digestive distress.

1 teaspoon olive oil	2 cups watercress leaves
2 leeks, topped, tailed, and chopped	4 scallions, minced
3 cups vegetable stock	1 cup skim milk or low-fat soy milk
2 cups fresh spinach, chopped	Pinch of sea salt

If the weather is damp: Add 1 or 2 cloves of minced garlic when you add the leeks.

If the weather is dry: Garnish with minced fresh cilantro before serving.

Heat a soup pot on medium-high and warm the oil. Add the leeks and sauté until fragrant and tender, 6 to 7 minutes. Pour in the stock and bring it to a boil. Reduce the heat to medium and toss in the spinach and cress, simmering until the greens are just wilted, 2 to 3 minutes.

Turn off the heat and let the soup relax for a couple of minutes, then pour it into a food processor or blender along with the scallions, milk, and salt, and process until the soup is smooth but still flecked with green. Serve warm for lunch or dinner, or pour into a Thermos to take to work or a picnic.

MAKES 4 SERVINGS; 75 CALORIES PER SERVING; 1 GRAM OF FAT; 12 PERCENT OF CALORIES FROM FAT.

watercress salad with artichokes and balsamic vinaigrette

If the weather is damp: Whisk in a pinch of white horseradish when preparing the dressing.

If the weather is dry: Serve juicy orange sections for dessert.

Cress provides vitamin C and beta carotene, for spring lung and skin health. In addition, the artichokes are moist and hydrating to refresh the system after a cold winter and exposure to dry indoor heat.

1 tablespoon balsamic vinegar
1 teaspoon prepared mustard
1 teaspoon olive oil
Pinch of sea salt
Freshly ground black pepper to taste

1 cup romaine lettuce hearts, coarsely chopped
2 cups watercress leaves
2 cups chopped cooked artichoke hearts (frozen or canned)

In a small bowl, whisk together the vinegar, mustard, olive oil, salt, and pepper.

In a serving bowl, combine the romaine, cress, and artichoke hearts. Pour on the dressing and toss well to combine. Serve with crusty whole grain bread as a light entrée for brunch, lunch, or dinner.

MAKES 4 SERVINGS; 67 CALORIES PER SERVING; 1 GRAM OF FAT; 14 PERCENT OF CALORIES FROM FAT.

spring greens with fresh herb dressing

The tarragon and dill in the dressing contain aromatic compounds that help keep digestion cool and fresh as the weather begins to heat up.

1 cup watercress leaves

2 cups fresh spinach leaves

3 cups spring mix, combining
   mustard greens, mizuna, frisée,
   radicchio, or your choice

1 scallion, coarsely chopped

¼ cup plain nonfat yogurt or soy
   yogurt

1 tablespoon minced fresh tarragon

1 tablespoon minced fresh dillweed

I tablespoon minced fresh chives

2 tablespoons lemon juice

1 teaspoon olive oil

Pinch of sea salt

If the weather is damp: Add a clove of minced garlic to the dressing.

If the weather is dry: Serve with slightly chilled peppermint tea.

In a salad bowl, combine the cress, spinach, and spring mix.

In a blender or food processor, combine the remaining ingredients and blend until smooth. Pour over the greens, tossing about 30 times to combine. Serve as an appetizer or as a side dish for lunch or dinner.

MAKES 4 SERVINGS; 51 CALORIES PER SERVING; 1 GRAM OF FAT; 18 PERCENT OF CALORIES FROM FAT.

mustard greens salad, vietnamese style

If the weather is damp: Be liberal with the hot pepper sauce.

If the weather is dry: Serve with lime wedges for drizzling.

These spring greens are a good source of magnesium, a mineral whose absence in the diet may cause spring headaches and irritability.

1 teaspoon prepared mustard
1 teaspoon hot pepper sauce, or to taste
1 teaspoon toasted (dark) sesame oil
2 tablespoons rice vinegar

1 teaspoon regular or reduced-sodium soy sauce
8 cups fresh mustard greens

In a large salad bowl, combine the prepared mustard, hot pepper sauce, sesame oil, vinegar, and soy sauce.

Arrange the mustard greens in a large strainer or colander. Pour boiling water over them for about 5 seconds. Pat the greens dry and tip them into the waiting bowl. Toss well to combine, about 30 times. Traditionally, this is a lunch entrée salad, but I like it for dinner, too.

MAKES 4 SERVINGS; 62 CALORIES PER SERVING; 1 GRAM OF FAT; 15 PERCENT OF CALORIES FROM FAT.

elbows with arugula

If the weather is damp: Add cayenne to taste when tossing.

If the weather is dry: Serve with lemonade as the beverage.

Arugula, a delicate member of the mustard family, is often recommended by herbalists as a mild spring diuretic.

2 cups arugula leaves
1 tablespoon olive oil
¼ cup minced fresh basil

Pinch of sea salt
Freshly ground black pepper to taste
4 cups hot, cooked elbow pasta

In a large bowl, combine all of the ingredients and toss well, about 30 times, until the arugula has just wilted. Serve warm as a lunch or dinner entrée.

MAKES 4 SERVINGS; 242 CALORIES PER SERVING; 4.5 GRAMS OF FAT; 17 PERCENT OF CALORIES FROM FAT.

dandelion vinegar

This tasty condiment is a good source of calcium, a mineral that can promote nerve health, strong bones, and fit teeth.

About 2 cups fresh dandelion leaves, coarsely chopped

Cider vinegar to cover (about 2½ cups)

Pack the dandelion leaves in a large glass jar and pour on vinegar to cover. Cover the jar and set it in a sunny window for about 2 weeks, shaking the jar once daily. After 2 weeks, discard the dandelion leaves and enjoy the vinegar in salads, soups, sauces, or marinades.

MAKES ABOUT 2 CUPS VINEGAR, OR THIRTY-TWO 1-TABLESPOON SERVINGS; LESS THAN 1 CALORIE PER SERVING; NO ADDED FAT.

If the weather is damp: Mince fresh jalapeños and let them marinate in the vinegar, to cover, for an hour before using to garnish a spring salad.

If the weather is dry: Fill a glass with half orange juice and half soda water, then swirl in half a teaspoon of the vinegar.

sprouts: seeds of good nutrition

Outside the gates of a rubber plantation near Kuala Lumpur, Malaysia, I stopped to look at a roadside Buddhist shrine whose sole ornamentation was a carved wooden plaque with a roundish design in the center. The design, I discovered later, is a symbol for the "seed of awakening," and the sprouting, so to speak, of all things new. How like spring, I thought, and what an interesting perspective to see every day with sproutlike enthusiasm.

Sprouts—the seeds of beans and vegetables, like radishes, that have begun to grow—are the quintessential spring food. They're fresh and nutritious, containing protein, stress-soothing B vitamins, beta carotene for lung and skin health, vitamin E for skin and heart health, and vitamin C for infection protection. Furthermore, one cup of sprouts contains less than 40 calories and virtually no fat.

To grow your own sprouts, start with seeds that are free from chemicals and pesticides. Soak about two tablespoons of the seeds in water overnight. Then rinse the seeds and set them in a quart-sized glass jar fitted with a special sprouting lid (available at natural food stores) or covered by cheesecloth fastened with a rubber band. Set the jar on its side, rinsing and draining the sprouts two to three times a day until they're one to two inches long. This will take about four days, but the time will vary slightly according to the type and size of the seeds you use, as well as the temperature of the room. On the last day of sprouting, put the seeds near a window so the little leaves will turn green with nutritious chlorophyll. Store the sprouts, covered and refrigerated, for up to a week.

quick cooking tips for sprouts

Seed sprouts, such as alfalfa, clover, radish, and sunflower, can be eaten raw in salads and in sandwiches, or used as an edible lining for serving platters. Sprouts from beans, such as mung, lentil, soy, and adzuki, should be lightly cooked for the best digestibility. Toss them into hot soup just before eating, and add them to a stir-fry or omelet during the last 30 seconds of cooking.

salmon salad with sprouts and ginger-lime dressing

If the weather is damp:
Add freshly ground pepper
to taste to the dressing
and serve the salad at
room temperature.

If the weather is dry: Serve
the salad slightly chilled.

This recipe is a tonic for spring sinus trouble, since the gingerroot may help clear the head. In addition, for those who become queasy when plagued with sinus congestion, gingerroot may help alleviate the problem.

2 cups shredded romaine lettuce

1½ cups radish sprouts, or other sprouts

12 ounces salmon fillet, cooked and loosely broken into pieces

1 teaspoon olive oil

Juice from 1 lime

2 teaspoons honey

1 teaspoon regular or reduced-sodium soy sauce

1 tablespoon finely grated fresh gingerroot

In a large bowl, combine the romaine, sprouts, and salmon.

In a small bowl, whisk together the remaining ingredients. Pour over the salad and toss well to combine, taking care not to break up the salmon pieces. Serve as a brunch, lunch, or dinner entrée salad.

MAKES 4 SERVINGS; 200 CALORIES PER SERVING; 6 GRAMS OF FAT; 27 PERCENT OF CALORIES FROM FAT.

green beans
myths and minerals

When a hairstylist told me that my hair grows so fast because I frequently eat green beans, I investigated and discovered that he may be right. The tasty and slender pods contain a compound called inositol, which indeed promotes hair growth. It also helps prevent hardening of the arteries and aids liver health. In addition, green beans are a decent nonmeat source of iron, especially when eaten with foods high in vitamin C, to assist absorption.

Curiously, this nutritious and very common vegetable is the source of lofty myths. Ancient Greeks and Romans spat beans at ghosts to scare them back to heaven. The Japanese, too, used beans to chase away evil spirits by scattering them around the house on the final day of winter. And then there is the universal Jack and the Bean Stalk fable. The stalk, symbolizing the ladder to heaven, corresponds with the rope trick of India; Jacob's ladder in the Middle East; and the New Guinea tale of Tauni-kapi-kapi, where a man and his mother climb a bean stalk to destroy an evil giant.

On a more pragmatic note, a cup of cooked green beans offers 125 calories and virtually no fat. Moreover, green beans are a good source of beta carotene, which helps promote healthy skin and lungs.

the bean family

Green beans come from the same plant as dried beans, but green beans are the infant, tender stage. As the pods grow, so do the seeds inside, and those seeds, when dried, are dried beans.

quick cooking tip for green beans

Steam topped and tailed green beans over boiling water until tender, checking at two-minute intervals for very small beans, and at four minutes and more for larger, tougher beans. Plan on about a pound of beans to serve four people, and toss them, warm, with fresh lemon juice and olive oil; or with chili oil and toasted chopped peanuts.

green beans with toasted sesame seeds and scallions

If the weather is damp: Stir in a clove of minced garlic when tossing with the sesame seeds.

If the weather is dry: Double the lemon juice and serve the green beans at room temperature or very slightly chilled.

The folk medicine of both Germany and France claims that a steady diet of green beans can soothe the pain of gout and rheumatism.

1 pound green beans

1 tablespoon sesame seeds

1 tablespoon balsamic vinegar

1 teaspoon regular or reduced-sodium soy sauce

1 tablespoon lemon juice

2 scallions, minced

Bring a pot of water to a boil and steam the green beans over the boiling water until they are bright green and just tender, about 4 minutes, depending on their size.

Meanwhile, in a sauté pan over medium-high heat, add the sesame seeds and stir constantly until toasted, about 2 minutes. When the green beans are ready, pat them dry and toss with the sesame seeds, vinegar, soy sauce, lemon juice, and scallions. Serve warm or at room temperature as a lunch or dinner side dish.

MAKES 4 SERVINGS; 80 CALORIES PER SERVING; 3 GRAMS OF FAT; 33 PERCENT OF CALORIES FROM FAT.

green beans with fresh oregano

Oregano offers aromatic compounds that help prevent spring indigestion.

1 pound green beans
1 ripe tomato, finely chopped,
   including juice
2 teaspoons red wine vinegar

1 clove garlic, minced
1 tablespoon minced fresh oregano
Pinch of sea salt

Steam the green beans over boiling water until they're bright green and just tender, about 4 minutes. Pat dry and toss immediately with the remaining ingredients. Serve warm or at room temperature as a lunch or dinner side dish.

MAKES 4 SERVINGS; 62 CALORIES PER SERVING; NO ADDED FAT.

If the weather is damp: Increase the garlic to 2 cloves, and sprinkle with freshly ground pepper before serving warm.

If the weather is dry: Substitute lemon juice for the vinegar, and serve the green beans at room temperature or very slightly chilled.

green beans with tomato and fresh spring herbs

The fragrance and texture of this dish are both refreshing and hydrating. In addition, the combination of thyme, tarragon, and dillweed makes it a digestive tonic.

1 pound green beans
1 large tomato, peeled and chopped
1 tablespoon white wine vinegar
1 teaspoon minced fresh thyme

1 teaspoon minced fresh tarragon
1 teaspoon minced fresh dillweed
Pinch of sea salt

Steam the green beans over boiling water until they're bright green and just tender, about 4 minutes.

Meanwhile, in a blender or food processor, combine the tomato, vinegar, thyme, tarragon, dill, and salt and process until smooth. When the green beans are done, pat them dry and toss with the tomato mixture. Serve warm or at room temperature as a lunch or dinner salad or side dish.

MAKES 4 SERVINGS; 67 CALORIES PER SERVING; NO ADDED FAT.

If the weather is damp: Add hot pepper sauce to taste before blending.

If the weather is dry: Serve the green beans slightly chilled on a bed of crisp spring greens.

green beans in garlic marinade

If the weather is damp:
Add hot pepper sauce to
taste to the marinade.

If the weather is dry:
Increase the lemon juice
to ¼ cup.

Garlic contains immune-boosting compounds that, when consumed daily, may help prevent spring sinus trouble and allergies.

¾ pound green beans

2 carrots, julienned

3 cloves garlic, minced

1 teaspoon dark (toasted) sesame oil

2 tablespoons balsamic vinegar

2 teaspoons lemon juice

1 teaspoon regular or reduced-
  sodium soy sauce

1 tablespoon minced fresh chives

Steam the green beans and carrots over boiling water until they're brightly colored and just tender, 3 to 4 minutes.

Meanwhile, in a medium bowl, whisk together the remaining ingredients. When the green beans and carrots are ready, pat them dry and add them to the bowl, tossing well to combine. Cover the bowl and refrigerate for at least 4 hours, or overnight. Serve very slightly chilled as a lunch or dinner salad.

MAKES 4 SERVINGS; 70 CALORIES PER SERVING; 1 GRAM OF FAT; 13 PERCENT OF CALORIES FROM FAT.

dill-simmered green beans with toasted almonds

The aromatics carvone and limonene make dillweed an excellent spring digestive tonic.

2 cups vegetable stock
Two 4–inch sprigs fresh dillweed
2 cloves garlic, halved
3 lemon slices

1 pound green beans
1 tablespoon slivered almonds
Pinch of sea salt

*If the weather is damp:
Add freshly ground black
pepper to taste when you
add the salt.*

*If the weather is dry:
Sprinkle with lemon juice
when you toss with the
almonds.*

In a frying pan on medium-high heat, bring the stock, dillweed, garlic, and
lemon to a simmer. Add the green beans, cover loosely, and continue to simmer
until the beans are bright green and tender, 3 to 4 minutes.

Meanwhile, heat a dry sauté pan on medium-high, and add the almonds, stirring constantly until they're toasted, about 2 minutes. When the green beans
are ready, drain them and toss with the almonds and salt. Serve warm or at
room temperature as a lunch or dinner side dish that's especially compatible
with grilled fish.

MAKES 4 SERVINGS; 60 CALORIES PER SERVING; TRACE OF FAT.

green beans with lemon-rosemary sauce

If the weather is damp: Increase the mustard to 2 teaspoons.

If the weather is dry: Serve at room temperature or very slightly chilled on a nest of crisp spring greens.

In parts of France and Germany, lemon is ingested daily to strengthen immunities and to help prevent spring flu.

1 pound green beans
1 shallot, minced
¼ cup vegetable stock
2 tablespoons lemon juice

One 2-inch sprig fresh rosemary
1½ teaspoons prepared mustard
1 teaspoon olive oil

Steam the green beans and the shallot over boiling water until they're tender, about 4 minutes. Meanwhile, in a small sauté pan, combine the stock, lemon juice, and rosemary, and bring to a boil. Whisk in the mustard and olive oil, continuing to whisk until the sauce has been reduced to about ¼ cup, about 2 minutes. Discard the rosemary. When the beans are ready, toss with the sauce and serve warm as an appetizer salad for lunch or dinner.

MAKES 4 SERVINGS; 77 CALORIES PER SERVING; 1 GRAM OF FAT; 12 PERCENT OF CALORIES FROM FAT.

green beans with hazelnut oil and fresh thyme

If the weather is damp: Add freshly ground black pepper when you add the sea salt.

If the weather is dry: Serve the beans drizzled with fresh lemon juice.

French herbalists recommend thyme to help prevent spring flu, because its main volatile oil, thymol, is anti-infective.

1 pound green beans
¼ cup vegetable stock
Five 1-inch sprigs thyme

1 teaspoon hazelnut oil
Pinch of sea salt

Steam the green beans over boiling water until they're bright green and just tender, about 4 minutes.

Meanwhile, in a small sauté pan boil the stock and thyme, stirring frequently, until the liquid has been reduced to about 1 tablespoon, about 2½ minutes. Discard the thyme, add the oil and salt, and toss with the green beans. Serve warm as a lunch or dinner side dish.

MAKES 4 SERVINGS; 70 CALORIES PER SERVING; 1 GRAM OF FAT; 13 PERCENT OF CALORIES FROM FAT.

stir-fried green beans with hot peppers and peanuts

This recipe is perfect for a chilly spring day, since the hot peppers and garlic increase circulation, thus warming the body.

1 pound green beans

1 teaspoon chili oil

1 teaspoon regular or reduced-
    sodium soy sauce

2 cloves garlic, minced

Three 2-inch dried hot peppers

2 tablespoons chopped peanuts

If the weather is damp:
Add hot pepper sauce to
taste when stir-frying, and
serve the dish warm.

If the weather is dry:
Serve very slightly chilled,
drizzled with lime juice.

Set the green beans in a strainer and pour boiling water over them for about 10 seconds. Pat them dry and set aside.

Heat a wok or large sauté pan on medium-high, then add the remaining ingredients and the beans. Stir-fry until they are fragrant, about 1 minute. Serve warm as a lunch or dinner side dish; or toss with 2 cups thin, just-cooked Chinese noodles and serve as an entrée.

MAKES 4 SERVINGS; 85 CALORIES PER SERVING; 3 GRAMS OF FAT; 31 PERCENT OF CALORIES FROM FAT.

green beans with garlic and spring sage

If the weather is damp:
Use cayenne instead of
black pepper.

If the weather is dry:
Serve chilled fresh orange
sections for dessert.

In England, where sage is called "red sage," herbalists recommend it to treat spring dyspepsia.

1 pound green beans	Pinch of sea salt
1 teaspoon olive oil	Freshly ground black pepper
1 clove garlic, minced	1 tablespoon balsamic vinegar
7 fresh sage leaves	

Steam the green beans over boiling water until they're bright green and just tender, about 4 minutes.

Meanwhile, in a small sauté pan, heat the olive oil, garlic, sage, salt, and pepper on medium-high for about 1 minute, or until the sage and garlic are fragrant. When the beans are done, pat them dry and toss with the garlic-sage mixture and the vinegar. Serve warm or at room temperature as a lunch or dinner side dish. Or serve slightly chilled atop crisp greens as an entrée salad.

MAKES 4 SERVINGS; 60 CALORIES PER SERVING; 1 GRAM OF FAT; 15 PERCENT OF CALORIES FROM FAT.

warm potato salad with green beans and basil

Basil is prescribed by English herbalists as an antispasmodic, a substance that treats stomach cramps and gas.

½ pound new potatoes, cut into
   1–inch pieces
½ pound green beans
1 tablespoons fresh basil leaves
1 shallot, minced

1 tablespoon cider vinegar
1 teaspoon olive oil
3 tablespoons buttermilk
Pinch of sea salt
Freshly ground black pepper

If the weather is damp:
Serve with a beverage of
spicy tomato juice.

If the weather is dry:
Serve with chilled
peppermint tea.

Steam the potatoes over boiling water until they're half-tender, about 4 minutes. Then add the green beans and continue to steam them until they're tender, about 4 minutes more.

Meanwhile, to a processor or blender, add the remaining ingredients and process until they're combined. When the potatoes and green beans are ready, pat them dry and toss with the basil mixture. Serve warm as a lunch or dinner entrée, with a side dish of vegetable soup.

MAKES 4 SERVINGS; 85 CALORIES PER SERVING; 1 GRAM OF FAT; 11 PERCENT OF CALORIES FROM FAT.

tuna salad with green beans and red wine–tarragon vinaigrette

If the weather is damp: Be liberal with the black pepper.

If the weather is dry: Add an extra tomato.

This crisp and hydrating salad is a refresher for those who are fatigued from stress and overwork, because tuna helps the brain produce the energizing hormone dopamine.

8 crisp romaine lettuce leaves
12 ounces tuna, packed in water
2 medium potatoes, cut into chunks
   and steamed
½ pound green beans, steamed
1 large, ripe tomato, cut into wedges
4 Greek olives, pitted and sliced

1 tablespoon red wine vinegar
1 tablespoon lemon juice
1 teaspoon olive oil
1 tablespoon minced fresh tarragon
Pinch of dried mustard
Pinch of sea salt
Freshly ground black pepper

Arrange the salad by placing the romaine leaves in a starburst pattern on a round platter. Mound the tuna in the center and fill in with the potatoes, green beans, and tomato. Sprinkle the olives over all.

In a small bowl, whisk together the remaining ingredients and sprinkle on the salad. Serve as a lunch or dinner entrée.

MAKES 4 SERVINGS; 177 CALORIES PER SERVING; 4 GRAMS OF FAT; 20 PERCENT OF CALORIES FROM FAT.

peas
nutrition to please

Up three flights of stairs through the red door facing east, I ventured in to talk with an elderly woman from China who had grown peas every spring for nearly seventy years. They're the first seeds in the ground, she told me. Plant them just as soon as the ground can be worked. It's very lucky, she continued, to plant peas on February 17, since in China pea blossoms are the birthday flower of that day, symbolizing great respect and happiness.

Westerners, too, are happy with peas, consuming millions of pounds annually. The most popular are the smooth, round, sweet peas that are shelled from pods, commonly called "garden" peas, or "English" peas. Edible-podded varieties, such as snap peas and snow peas, are more popular in China, but are gaining favor here, too. Both types are low in calories (125 calories per cup for garden peas; 65 calories per cup for edible pods); low in fat; and offer modest amounts of calcium for strong bones and nerves, iron to fight fatigue, beta carotene for skin and lung health, and potassium to support normal blood pressure levels. In addition, peas are a good source of nonmeat protein and of insoluble fiber, which promotes digestive health and aids in weight loss.

flower power

Pea blossoms are edible, delicate white flowers that make beautiful garnishes for spring salads.

quick cooking tips for peas

Some edible-podded peas may need to be destrung before cooking. To do so, pinch the stem string of a pea with your thumb and index finger, and zip it down and off. Both edible-podded and garden peas can easily be steamed, but start checking edible-podded varieties for doneness after one minute. Garden peas may take four minutes to steam. Toss a quarter cup of any variety of steamed peas into the batter for an omelet to serve two, or into potato salad for two.

bulgur with lemon, parsley, and fresh peas

If the weather is damp: Add freshly ground pepper to taste when you add the salt.

If the weather is dry: Serve on a nest of crisp spring greens.

The wheat in this salad is a good source of calming B vitamins, which help soothe spring stresses. It also offers some insoluble fiber, a plus for healthy digestion.

½ cup bulgur
½ cup hot vegetable stock
Juice from 1 lemon
1 cup fresh green peas

½ cup chopped fresh parsley leaves
1 carrot, julienned
1 tablespoon olive oil
Pinch of sea salt

In a bowl, combine the bulgur, stock, and lemon juice and let the bulgur soak until all of the liquid has been absorbed, about 20 minutes.

Meanwhile, in a small saucepan, simmer the peas in about an inch of water until bright green and just tender, about 3 minutes. Drain, toss the bulgur with the peas, parsley, carrot, oil, and salt, and serve warm, at room temperature, or very slightly chilled as a lunch or dinner entrée. Or use as a stuffing for steamed whole artichokes.

MAKES 4 SERVINGS; 155 CALORIES PER SERVING; 4 GRAMS OF FAT; 23 PERCENT OF CALORIES FROM FAT.

ginger-simmered peas

Gingerroot, rich in stomach-soothing volatile oils, can help avert spring bloat and indigestion.

¼ cup vegetable stock

1 clove garlic, sliced

1 teaspoon regular or
   reduced-sodium soy sauce

3 slices fresh gingerroot

1 pound snow peas, strings removed

In a medium sauté pan, heat the stock, garlic, soy sauce, and gingerroot on medium-high heat. Add the snow peas and cook them, stirring constantly, until they are bright green and just tender, about 1 minute. Drain the peas, discard the garlic and gingerroot, and serve warm, at room temperature, or very slightly chilled as a side dish; or toss with hot rice and serve as an entrée with a side of steamed vegetables.

MAKES 4 SERVINGS; 72 CALORIES PER SERVING; NO ADDED FAT.

If the weather is damp: Increase the gingerroot to 5 slices.

If the weather is dry: Add a slice of lemon to the stock before cooking the peas.

peas with shallots and fresh tarragon

As a spring tonic for water retention, tarragon acts as a mild diuretic.

½ cup vegetable stock

1 bay leaf

2 cups fresh green peas

1 shallot, minced

1 tablespoon minced fresh tarragon

Pinch of sea salt

In a saucepan, bring the stock and bay leaf to a boil on high heat. Add the peas and shallot and continue to boil until the peas are bright green and just tender, 3 to 5 minutes. Drain (don't lose the shallot) and toss with the tarragon and salt. Serve warm as a side dish.

MAKES 4 SERVINGS; 40 CALORIES PER SERVING; NO ADDED FAT.

If the weather is damp: Add freshly ground pepper to taste when you add the salt.

If the weather is dry: Serve chilled peppermint tea with the meal.

rice cakes with spring peas

If the weather is damp: Serve the cakes with spicy salsa.

If the weather is dry: Serve the cakes with lemon wedges for drizzling.

These light, savory cakes make a rejuvenating spring repast, combining chives, parsley, and basil to entice your taste buds out of their winter doldrums.

1 cup fresh green peas
3 cups cooked short-grain rice, such as arborio, at room temperature
4 egg whites
1 tablespoon minced fresh chives
1 tablespoon minced fresh parsley

1 tablespoon minced fresh basil
1 tablespoon grated Parmesan cheese or soy Parmesan
About ½ cup fine whole wheat bread crumbs
2 teaspoons olive oil

Blanch the peas by placing them in a strainer and pouring boiling water over them for about 10 seconds. Combine the peas with the rice, egg whites, chives, parsley, basil, and Parmesan. Divide the mixture into sixths, forming each portion into a very firm ball, then into a little cake. Press each cake lightly on both sides in the bread crumbs, then brush each side lightly with the oil.

Broil the cakes about 4 inches from the heat source until they are lightly browned, about 2 minutes on each side. Serve warm as a lunch or dinner entrée in place of fatty, meat-based burgers.

MAKES 6 CAKES; 180 CALORIES PER CAKE; 2 GRAMS OF FAT; 10 PERCENT OF CALORIES FROM FAT.

peas with garlic, cress, and dill

A tonifying trio, garlic, watercress, and dillweed will revive your mood with spring freshness. They will also aid digestion, due to the aromatic compounds they contain.

1 teaspoon olive oil
2 cloves garlic, minced
2 teaspoons minced fresh dillweed
2 cups fresh green peas

1 cup watercress leaves
Pinch of sea salt
Freshly ground black pepper to taste

If the weather is damp: Be liberal with the black pepper.

If the weather is dry: Add 1 teaspoon lemon juice while sautéing.

Heat a sauté pan on medium-high, and add the oil. When the oil is warm, add the garlic, dillweed, and peas, and sauté until the peas have begun to turn bright green, about 2 minutes. Toss in the watercress and sauté for about 20 seconds more. Season with salt and pepper. Serve warm as a side dish; or slightly chilled as a side salad.

MAKES 4 SERVINGS; 82 CALORIES PER SERVING; 1 GRAM OF FAT; 12 PERCENT OF CALORIES FROM FAT.

pea and scallion won tons

If the weather is damp:
Serve the won tons with
prepared mustard, or make
a dipping sauce of ¹/₄ cup
soy sauce with wasabe
horseradish stirred in to
taste.

If the weather is dry: Serve
the won tons with a
dipping sauce of ¹/₄ cup
soy sauce mixed with
toasted (dark) sesame oil
and lemon juice to taste.

Scallions help to stimulate the appetite and promote good digestion.

³/₄ **cup fresh green peas**
¹/₂ **cup minced scallions**

20 round won ton wrappers (available in the frozen foods section at Asian markets and many supermarkets—buy the ones containing no preservatives)

In a small bowl, combine the peas and scallions. To make a won ton, set a wrapper on the counter, or on a won ton press, which looks like a set of false teeth and is available at Asian markets. Dip a finger in water and run it all along the outer edge of the won ton. Set about a tablespoon of the pea mixture in the center, fold the won ton in half, and press the edges tight with the tines of a fork. If you are using a won ton press, just fold it over on itself and press. Repeat with all of the won tons.

In a large frying pan, simmer, but don't boil, about 2 inches of water. Use a slotted spoon to set the won tons into the water. Don't crowd them. Let them simmer gently for about 1 minute, or until they float, and you can see the peas turning a brighter green inside. Serve warm as an appetizer or entrée.

MAKES 20 WON TONS, OR 4 SERVINGS; 125 CALORIES PER SERVING; NO ADDED FAT.

peas with mustard-sage vinaigrette

Mustard and watercress are good sources of the mineral magnesium, which helps to promote a balanced spring disposition.

2 cups cooked fresh green peas
1 cup finely minced watercress
   leaves
1 carrot, grated
2 tablespoons lemon juice

1 teaspoon balsamic vinegar
1 teaspoon minced fresh sage
2 teaspoons olive oil
1 teaspoon prepared mustard
Pinch of sea salt

If the weather is damp: Add freshly ground pepper when you add the salt.

If the weather is dry: Serve on a nest of crisp romaine lettuce.

In a medium bowl, combine the peas, cress, and carrot. In a small bowl, combine the lemon juice, vinegar, sage, olive oil, mustard, and salt. Pour the vinaigrette over the pea mixture and toss well to combine. Serve as a side dish or salad.

MAKES 4 SERVINGS; 72 CALORIES PER SERVING; 1 GRAM OF FAT; 13 PERCENT OF CALORIES FROM FAT.

snow peas with sesame and orange zest

The uplifting aroma of orange gives a springlike spin to this dish. The carrots offer beta carotene, promoting good spring skin health.

4 cups snow peas, strings removed
1 carrot, julienned
½ teaspoon orange zest

1 teaspoon toasted (dark) sesame oil
1 teaspoon regular or reduced-
   sodium soy sauce

If the weather is damp: Add hot pepper sauce to taste.

If the weather is dry: Add fresh lemon juice to taste.

Set the peas and carrot in a large strainer and blanch them by pouring boiling water over them for about 10 seconds. Tip them into a medium bowl and add the zest, sesame oil, and soy sauce, stirring well to combine. Serve warm or at room temperature as a side dish or salad.

MAKES 4 SERVINGS; 116 CALORIES PER SERVING; 1 GRAM OF FAT; 8 PERCENT OF CALORIES FROM FAT.

asparagus
spears for stamina

One steamy April in Kuala Lumpur, Malaysia, I learned to cook asparagus the *nonyo* way, a culinary style combining Chinese and Southeast Asian techniques. As instructed, I simmered about an inch of water in a large frying pan, then laid a thick chopstick in the bottom, near the edge of the pan. I set the asparagus in, resting the buds in a row on the chopstick, elevating them above the water to prevent their overcooking. The spears simmered, loosely covered, until they were bright green and just tender, about four minutes (thick spears will take longer). Drizzled with lemon juice, salt, and peanut oil, the dish was deliciously reviving.

One reason my Malaysian asparagus—and other asparagus preparations, for that matter—may renew the spirits is that asparagus is an excellent source of the nutrient folate, which helps restore energy. Folate may also help abate depression and anxiety; and it is critical in pregnancy to assure healthy fetal development. Asparagus is also a good source of cancer-fighting vitamin C, beta carotene, and selenium, and it contains traces of iron, potassium, and riboflavin—a B vitamin that aids the body in absorbing other nerve-soothing B vitamins. For all that good nutrition, half a cup of cooked asparagus contains 23 calories and virtually no fat.

An hour or so after eating asparagus, many people notice their urine smells peculiar. It's merely a harmless sulfur compound, and not a permanent condition.

quick cooking tips for asparagus

In addition to the Malaysian method, one easy way to prepare asparagus is in the microwave. First hold each spear in both hands and snap off and discard the tough part. If the spears are thick, use a swivel-bladed vegetable peeler to peel the spears, leaving on a slice of peel here and there for color. Arrange the spears on a flat plate in a starburst design with the tender tips at the center, and cover with vented plastic wrap. For a pound of asparagus, microwave on full power for four to five minutes, depending on the thickness of the spears. Let the spears relax for about two minutes before enjoying in salads, or combined with sautéed mushrooms and dressed with lemon juice and olive oil. Or as a friend suggests, toss with minced scallion, minced red and yellow bell peppers, and a splash of balsamic vinegar. Then chill.

bay-steamed asparagus

*If the weather is damp:
Serve the spears warm,
and sprinkle with freshly
ground pepper when you
add the salt.*

*If the weather is dry: Serve
the spears slightly chilled.*

In China I learned a tip for maximizing the flavor of asparagus—cut it on a severe diagonal before cooking. Exposing more surface area reveals more flavor, as you will note in the bay-scented morsels that follow.

3 bay leaves
1 pound asparagus spears, trimmed
   and cut on a severe diagonal
1 shallot, minced

Juice of 1 lemon
1 tablespoon minced fresh parsley
Pinch of sea salt

Add the bay leaves to a medium pot containing several inches of boiling water. Set in a steamer basket and steam the asparagus and shallot, covered, until just tender, 3 to 4 minutes depending on the thickness and toughness of the spears. Pat the asparagus dry and toss with the lemon juice, parsley, and salt. Serve warm as a side dish, or tossed with 2 cups hot penne pasta as an entrée. Or chill the asparagus and serve as a salad tossed with watercress and curly red lettuce.

MAKES 4 SERVINGS; 30 CALORIES PER SERVING; NO ADDED FAT.

penne with garlic-simmered asparagus

Garlic is an effective spring tonic; its volatile oils are anti-infective, helping to prevent coughs, colds, flu, and other spring infections.

2 teaspoons olive oil
4 cloves garlic, thinly sliced
About ½ pound asparagus, sliced
   into 2-inch pieces
⅔ cup vegetable stock

2 cups cooked penne pasta
   (½ pound dried)
¼ cup grated Parmesan cheese or
   soy Parmesan

If the weather is damp: Add a pinch of cayenne when you add the Parmesan.

If the weather is dry: Add 1 teaspoon lemon juice to the stock before adding it to the pan.

Heat a large sauté pan on medium-high, then add the oil. When the oil is warm, add the garlic and asparagus and sauté for about 1 minute. Pour in the stock, cover loosely, and raise the heat to high, letting the mixture bubble until the asparagus is bright green and just tender, 3 to 4 minutes. Toss with the penne and sprinkle with the Parmesan. Serve warm as a lunch or dinner entrée.

MAKES 2 LARGE SERVINGS; 290 CALORIES PER SERVING; 8 GRAMS OF FAT; 25 PERCENT OF CALORIES FROM FAT.

couscous with asparagus and saffron

If the weather is damp:
Add hot pepper sauce to
taste when simmering the
tomato mixture.

If the weather is dry: Serve
with a salad of crisp
greens, tossed with a
lemony or other citrus-
based dressing.

East Indian Ayurvedic herbalists recommend saffron as a rejuvenative herb to treat such spring inflammatory conditions as asthma, cough, and irritable bowel syndrome.

1 tablespoon olive oil
1 leek, topped, tailed, and chopped
1 clove garlic, minced
1 large tomato, cored, seeded, and chopped
2 tablespoons golden raisins
1 cup chopped cooked asparagus

½ teaspoon ground cinnamon
½ teaspoon saffron threads, crushed
2 cups cooked whole wheat or white couscous
⅓ cup chopped fresh parsley
Pinch of sea salt

Heat a large sauté pan on medium-high, then add the oil. When the oil is warm, add the leek and garlic and sauté until fragrant and lightly browned, 4 to 5 minutes. Add the tomato, raisins, asparagus, cinnamon, and saffron, and continue to cook, stirring frequently, until the tomato has "melted" and the sauce is fragrant, about 5 minutes.

In a bowl, combine the tomato mixture with the couscous, parsley, and salt and toss well. Serve warm or at room temperature as a lunch or dinner entrée.

MAKES 2 LARGE SERVINGS; 305 CALORIES PER SERVING; 6 GRAMS OF FAT; 18 PERCENT OF CALORIES FROM FAT.

asparagus with honey-soy marinade

Chinese herbalists say that honey is cooling and soothing to a stressed body, and they recommend it daily in foods to treat fatigue and weakness.

1 pound asparagus
¼ cup rice vinegar
1 teaspoon toasted (dark) sesame oil
1 tablespoon honey

1 teaspoon regular or reduced-
   sodium soy sauce
1 teaspoon lemon juice

If the weather is damp: Add hot pepper sauce to taste to the marinade.

If the weather is dry: Top the marinating asparagus with 3 lemon slices.

Steam the asparagus spears over boiling water until they're bright green and tender, about 4 minutes. In a small bowl, combine the vinegar, sesame oil, honey, soy sauce, and lemon juice. When the spears are ready, arrange them in a shallow dish and pour on the marinade. Cover and chill for at least 3 hours, or as long as overnight. Serve slightly chilled as a salad or side dish.

MAKES 4 SERVINGS; 50 CALORIES PER SERVING; 1 GRAM OF FAT; 18 PERCENT OF CALORIES FROM FAT.

asparagus with lemon and chives

Fresh lemon juice, such as that which flavors this succulent asparagus dish, stimulates saliva production, thus improving digestion.

1 pound asparagus
Juice of 1 lemon

1 tablespoon minced fresh chives
Pinch of sea salt

If the weather is damp: Add a clove of minced fresh garlic when you add the lemon juice, and serve the asparagus warm.

If the weather is dry: Serve the asparagus slightly chilled, with lemon wedges for drizzling.

Steam the asparagus over boiling water until they're tender, about 4 minutes. Toss with the lemon juice, chives, and salt. Serve warm or very slightly chilled as a salad, appetizer, or side dish.

MAKES 4 SERVINGS; 33 CALORIES PER SERVING; NO ADDED FAT.

asparagus with citrus butter and fresh thyme

If the weather is damp:
Add freshly ground black
pepper to taste when you
add the salt.

———

If the weather is dry: Serve
the asparagus at room
temperature on a bed of
crisp spring greens.

Though butter in large amounts can deter good health, a small amount, such as that which is offered here, may be beneficial. Butter contains buteric acid, which helps the body absorb nutrients from food.

1 pound asparagus

2 teaspoons unsalted butter

¼ teaspoon grated orange peel

½ teaspoon minced fresh thyme

Pinch of sea salt

Steam the asparagus over boiling water until they're tender, about 4 minutes.

Meanwhile, in a small sauté pan over medium heat, combine the butter, orange peel, thyme, and salt, heating until the butter has melted, about 1½ minutes. When the asparagus is ready, toss it with the butter and serve warm or at room temperature as an appetizer or side dish.

MAKES 4 SERVINGS; 50 CALORIES PER SERVING; 2 GRAMS OF FAT; 35 PERCENT OF CALORIES FROM FAT.

wild rice salad with spring vegetables

Here is a spring festival in a meal, combining asparagus, peas, cress, and such spring herbs as parsley, chives, and thyme. The mild diuretic action of these delicious ingredients makes the dish a good spring tonic for those who have indulged in salty junk food.

1½ cups cooked brown or white rice

1½ cups cooked wild rice

1 pound asparagus, sliced into
   1-inch diagonals and cooked

4 scallions, minced

¼ cup minced fresh parsley

⅔ cup watercress leaves

¼ cup raisins

¼ cup fresh green peas

1 tablespoon olive oil

2 tablespoons rice vinegar

2 cloves garlic, minced

1 shallot, minced

1 teaspoon minced fresh chives

1 tablespoon minced fresh thyme

Pinch of saffron threads

Pinch of sea salt

If the weather is damp: Add hot pepper sauce to taste to the dressing before tossing with the rice.

If the weather is dry: Substitute 1 tablespoon lemon juice for 1 tablespoon of the vinegar.

In a large serving bowl, combine the rices, asparagus, scallions, parsley, cress, raisins, and peas.

In a small bowl, combine the remaining ingredients. Pour the dressing over the rice mixture and use a large rubber spatula to toss it all together, about 30 times. Serve as a lunch or dinner entrée with side dishes such as grilled zucchini and steamed snow peas.

MAKES 4 SERVINGS; 301 CALORIES PER SERVING; 3.5 GRAMS OF FAT; 11 PERCENT OF CALORIES FROM FAT.

radish
next-morning's nostrum

When a colleague overindulged in a meal of sake and greasy tempura, I observed as a Japanese herbalist created a remedy. He grated a daikon radish, then squeezed the gratings to make a juice. Adding a pinch of sea salt to the quarter cup of radish juice, the herbalist instructed my colleague, "Drink it, and your gallbladder will thank you."

Radish, it seems, is the universal cure-all for too much of whatever. I have seen radish juice with honey prescribed in Germany; in Italy radish juice is taken with olive oil; and in China it's radish juice with gingerroot juice. Tastewise, it's easy to see how the sharp flavor of radish would "cut" the lingering, heavy feeling of having overindulged. Herbalists say radish is a cholagogue; it tones and rebalances the liver and gallbladder. And, in fact, scientific research has determined that radishes contain erucic acid, which helps abate abdominal fullness and indigestion.

Other reasons to keep radishes on hand: They contain indoles, which are cancer-fighting compounds; vitamin C to help neutralize the ravages of spring stresses; folate for calm nerves; and raphanin, a natural anti-infective. Radishes are also a fine weight-loss food, containing only 10 calories for each half cup, and virtually no fat.

In the store you'll find small, round red radishes; long white daikon radishes sometimes the length of your arm; and black-skinned radishes the size of a turnip, which are popular in France and Germany. Herbalists agree that the three have equal healing benefits, so buy the ones that appeal to you.

✴ **quick cooking tips for radishes**

Grate or thinly slice raw radishes into green salads and marinated vegetable salads. Or dice radishes to add to soups and stir-fries in place of water chestnuts.

spicy marinated radish

In Hong Kong I learned to eat this pickle after meals, to encourage good digestion. It has a cleansing, refreshing taste and a crunchy texture.

½ pound daikon or other radish, julienned
1 carrot, julienned
¾ cup rice vinegar
Juice of 1 lemon
2 teaspoons honey

2 slices fresh gingerroot
2 cloves garlic, sliced
2 dried hot chile peppers
1 tablespoon minced lemongrass
1 tablespoon regular or reduced-sodium soy sauce

If the weather is damp: Munch on a serving as a midafternoon snack.

If the weather is dry: Add 3 lemon slices to the marinade before refrigerating.

Arrange the radish and carrot in a large glass bowl.

In a medium saucepan, combine the remaining ingredients and bring to a boil. Pour the mixture over the radish, cover, and let marinate, refrigerated, for at least 24 hours.

The radish will keep, covered and refrigerated, for up to 2 weeks. Serve as a condiment or relish with grilled fish, grilled vegetables, or sandwiches. Or add to green salads for an extra zip.

MAKES ABOUT 2 CUPS OR EIGHT ¼-CUP SERVINGS; 20 CALORIES PER SERVING; NO ADDED FAT.

crisp radish salad, malaysian style

If the weather is damp: Increase the garlic to 2 cloves.

This fresh and reviving dish reminds me of one I enjoyed at lunch in Port Dixon, Malaysia. We were served a lightly fried bass-type fish, cooked with garlic and chili paste, and the cool, fresh radish salad provided a wonderful balance.

If the weather is dry: Serve atop a nest of crisp greens.

2 cups sliced radishes
1 red bell pepper, seeded, cored, and sliced
2 scallions, minced

Juice of 1 lime
1 tablespoon regular or reduced-sodium soy sauce
1 clove garlic, minced

In a medium-sized bowl, combine all of the ingredients and toss well to combine. Serve at room temperature or very slightly chilled as a side dish to grilled fish, meat, or poultry.

MAKES 4 SERVINGS; 24 CALORIES PER SERVING; NO ADDED FAT.

japanese "salsa"

If the weather is damp: Add a sprinkle of freshly ground black pepper.

Once, at a lecture, just after I explained the digestive benefits of the pungent radish, a participant commented, "Oh, kind of like a Japanese salsa."

If the weather is dry: Add a couple of drops of lemon juice.

¼ cup grated radish

5 drops regular or reduced-sodium soy sauce

Mound the radish on a plate and sprinkle the soy sauce on top. Serve as an accompaniment to such fried foods as egg rolls, tempura, or fried fish.

MAKES 1 SERVING; 6 CALORIES PER SERVING; NO ADDED FAT.

strawberries
fruitful nutrition

One spring, with snow still on my boots, I created dozens of strawberry recipes for a magazine article I was writing. My kitchen filled with bowls and bowls of sweet red kisses. I baked shortcakes and tarts; froze ice cream and sorbet; mashed strawberries into mascarpone cheese to spread on morning muffins; marinated swordfish in a tart ginger-strawberry marinade; made strawberry butter for fresh berry pancakes; and whipped up strawberry mayonnaise for tea sandwiches.

Although my work was great fun, it was also nutritious, since strawberries are an excellent source of the "infection protection" nutrient, vitamin C. They are also a good source of dietary fiber, for healthy digestion; and a good source of ellagic acid, which has cancer-fighting properties. Furthermore, one cup of strawberries contains 45 calories and virtually no fat, making them a good snack for dieters.

sweet success

For the best-tasting strawberries, make sure they're ripe before you eat them. Ripe berries are shiny, and are a full, rich red. If your strawberries are not ripe, set them on a plate in a single layer and cover loosely with plastic wrap. Set the plate atop your refrigerator overnight, checking for ripeness in the morning.

quick cooking tip for strawberries

For the best flavor and maximum vitamin C content, it's best to eat strawberries uncooked. Enjoy them in a salad with arugula, toasted sesame seeds, and orange vinaigrette; tossed with sections of pink grapefruit and champagne vinegar; with cracked wheat, lemon juice, and fresh thyme. Or make strawberry ice cubes to chill refreshing spring beverages: Fill an ice cube tray halfway with water or orange juice and freeze. When frozen, set a small strawberry, or a strawberry slice, on each cube and fill the rest of the way with water or juice.

strawberry vinegar

If the weather is damp: Add 1 tablespoon of the strawberry vinegar to a spicy soup or chili to serve 4.

This fragrant condiment is based upon an old Austrian spring tonic that is said to strengthen and calm the entire nervous system. One way it may work is that strawberries are a good source of the nerve-soothing nutrient folate.

1 cup strawberries, sliced   **About 1 cup cider vinegar**

If the weather is dry: Mix ½ teaspoon of the vinegar in 1 cup of chilled seltzer water and sip.

Arrange the berries in a glass jar.

In a medium-sized saucepan, heat the vinegar until just warm. Don't boil. Pour the vinegar over the berries and let it cool for about 20 minutes. Then cover the jar and keep it in a sunny window for about a week, shaking the jar daily. Drain and discard the berries and use the vinegar in salad dressings, marinades, sauces, and soups, or to deglaze pans.

Or mix 2 tablespoons of the vinegar with ⅔ cup water and splash on the face as a skin toner or aftershave. Store the vinegar at room temperature; store the skin toner refrigerated.

MAKES 1 CUP, OR 16 1-TABLESPOON SERVINGS; LESS THAN 1 CALORIE PER SERVING; NO ADDED FAT.

fresh strawberry jam

For those with gout, this jam may help abate the pain, since strawberries contain blood-purifying compounds that help rid the body of uric acid.

2 cups strawberries, sliced   **2 tablespoons pure maple syrup**

In a large frying pan, combine the berries and the syrup and cook over medium-high heat, mashing the berries as they cook. Once the mixture is juicy, simmer, stirring frequently, until it's slightly thickened, about 7 minutes. Let the jam cool, then store covered and refrigerated for up to 2 weeks. Spread on toast, waffles, or scones; or swirl a spoonful into plain yogurt.

MAKES ABOUT 1½ CUPS, OR TWELVE 2-TABLESPOON SERVINGS; 15 CALORIES PER SERVING; NO ADDED FAT.

If the weather is damp: Spread the jam on warm cinnamon-apple muffins or scones.

If the weather is dry: Combine ¼ cup of the jam with ¼ cup orange juice and use as a glaze for grilled fresh pineapple.

strawberry-rhubarb dessert sauce

For those with sluggish spring digestion, this high-fiber dessert sauce will help provide relief. As when introducing any high-fiber food into the diet, be sure to drink eight 8-ounce glasses of water a day; otherwise, all that fiber could get "stuck."

1 cup strawberries, sliced   **¼ cup orange juice concentrate**
3 cups sliced rhubarb

In a large frying pan, combine all of the ingredients and heat on medium-high, mashing the fruit as you go, and bringing the mixture slowly to a boil as the juice is released. Reduce the heat to low and simmer slowly, stirring frequently, until the mixture looks slightly thickened and saucy, 15 to 20 minutes. Serve warm or chilled atop ice cream, frozen yogurt, cake, fruit salad, or crepes.

MAKES 2½ CUPS, OR FIVE ½-CUP SERVINGS; 50 CALORIES PER SERVING; NO ADDED FAT.

If the weather is damp: Add a pinch of ground cinnamon to the sauce while simmering.

If the weather is dry: Swirl in ½ teaspoon vanilla extract after simmering.

strawberries in balsamic vinegar

If the weather is damp: Serve the berries at room temperature and skip the mint.

If the weather is dry: Serve the berries slightly chilled.

When your berries are too tart, instead of adding sugar, try this refreshing spring dessert.

4 cups strawberries, sliced   4 sprigs fresh mint
1 tablespoon balsamic vinegar

In a medium bowl, toss the berries with the vinegar and let them relax for about 30 minutes. Then arrange the berries (including juice) in chilled dessert bowls, garnish with the mint, and serve as a dessert for brunch, lunch, or dinner.

MAKES 4 SERVINGS; 48 CALORIES PER SERVING; NO ADDED FAT.

lemon cake with fresh strawberries

This light spring dessert is a good source of digestion-toning fiber, an attribute many sweets lack.

3/4 cup whole wheat pastry flour
3/4 cup unbleached flour
12 egg whites, at room temperature
1 teaspoon cream of tartar
1½ teaspoons lemon extract
½ cup barley malt or honey
1 cup nonfat ricotta cheese or creamy-style soy cheese

1 cup nonfat vanilla yogurt or soy yogurt
1/3 cup orange juice concentrate
Pinch of sea salt
3 cups strawberries, sliced

If the weather is damp: *Serve with hot cinnamon-spice tea.*

If the weather is dry: *Serve with chilled peppermint tea.*

Preheat the oven to 325°F.

Into a bowl, sift the flours together, then return them to the sifter. In a large bowl, beat the egg whites, cream of tartar, and lemon extract on medium speed until the whites form soft peaks. Continue to beat the whites to stiff peaks while you add the barley malt or honey. Gradually sift ¼-cup measures of the flour mixture over the whites, folding in with a rubber spatula, until all of the flour has been incorporated.

Spoon the batter into a 9- or 10-inch removable-bottom tube pan and level off the top. Bake until the top is golden and springs back when you touch it, about 45 minutes. Then invert the pan on a wire rack and let it cool for about an hour.

Meanwhile, in a blender or food processor, combine the cheese, yogurt, juice concentrate, and salt and process until smooth and creamy. Then chill.

When the cake is ready, run a thin knife around the outside edge and remove the outer pan ring. Run a thin knife around the center tube and bottom of the cake. Slice the cake and serve with the ricotta mixture and strawberries atop.

MAKES 10 SERVINGS; 190 CALORIES PER SERVING; NO ADDED FAT.

fresh strawberry sherbet

If the weather is damp: Top each serving with a crunchy oat granola; or serve the sherbet atop waffles or in a crisp waffle cone.

If the weather is dry: Top each serving with fresh sliced strawberries.

Scientific researchers hold that eating strawberries may keep the heart healthy—the fruit contains a type of fiber that may help lower blood cholesterol levels.

4 cups strawberries   **2 egg whites, beaten to stiff peaks**

Toss the berries into a food processor or blender and process until pureed. Scoop the berries into a bowl and fold in the whites. Process the mixture in an ice cream maker according to the manufacturer's directions.

MAKES 4 LARGE SERVINGS; 60 CALORIES PER SERVING; NO ADDED FAT.

strawberry-orange milk shake

If the weather is damp: Add a pinch of freshly grated nutmeg before blending.

If the weather is dry: Instead of 2 cups milk, use 1 cup milk and 1 cup chilled orange juice.

For those who ban bran, this tasty shake will help fill the day's fiber requirements.

1 cup strawberries   **1 orange, peeled, seeded, and**
2 cups skim or soy milk, chilled   **separated into segments**

In a blender or food processor, combine all of the ingredients and blend until smooth. Serve immediately for breakfast, a snack, or dessert.

MAKES 2 SERVINGS; 122 CALORIES PER SERVING; NO ADDED FAT.

salmon
heart of good health

On a remote island in Puget Sound I watched as an Aleut Indian cook built a round, alderwood fire on which to smoke fresh salmon. He pressed long sticks into the ground vertically around the fire, then bound them together at the top. To each stick he tied a whole salmon that had been split down the middle to hang flat, then waited as the alder smoke cooked and seasoned the fish. Salmon, he explained, is a symbol of abundance and wisdom, and cooking it in the "old way" is a ceremony of sorts to honor those attributes.

In recent years, salmon has garnered even more accolades, especially for heart health. Research has shown that as few as two salmon meals a week—3.5 ounces each, about 185 calories—can help make blood less prone to the irregular clotting that can lead to a heart attack. In addition, salmon contains the omega type of oil that can help lower blood cholesterol levels. Add to that salmon's stroke-preventing potassium content, and we can see why the Aleut tribes believe that eating salmon is associated with wisdom.

quick cooking tips for salmon

To remove small bones from fillets, first run your hand against the grain of the flesh to find them, then pluck them out with tweezers. To cook salmon, paint fillets with a lemon vinaigrette and bake for about twenty minutes, or grill for eight to ten minutes, depending on the thickness of the fillets. Poach fillets in vegetable stock and herbs for about 10 minutes, then let the salmon cool (refrigerated) in the stock. Serve cold with prepared mustard, purple onion, and crusty bread.

salmon pâté with shallot and fresh parsley

If the weather is damp: Add a minced fresh jalapeño while mashing.

If the weather is dry: Add lemon juice to taste while mashing.

Those who experience "spring fever," or lack of energy, may wish to add salmon to their diets. The high protein content of the fish helps the brain release dopamine, an energizing hormone.

8 ounces cooked salmon
¼ cup plain nonfat yogurt or soy yogurt
¼ cup nonfat cream cheese or creamy soy cheese

1 shallot, minced
2 tablespoons minced fresh parsley
Pinch of sea salt

In a bowl, combine all of the ingredients and mash with a fork until the mixture is spreadable. Use as a sandwich spread; or serve as a snack or appetizer on cucumber rounds, crackers, or crusty bread.

MAKES 1½ CUPS, OR SIXTEEN 2–TABLESPOON SERVINGS; 40 CALORIES PER SERVING; 1.5 GRAMS OF FAT; 33 PERCENT OF CALORIES FROM FAT.

baked salmon with chiles and lime

This "packaged" method of cooking leaves the salmon moist and succulent without added fat and calories, making this a tasty and light spring meal.

12 ounces salmon fillet

2 jalapeño peppers, cored, seeded, and thinly sliced

2 cloves garlic, minced

Juice of 1 lime

Pinch of sea salt

1 lemon, sliced

If the weather is damp: Sprinkle on freshly ground black pepper to taste when you add the salt, and serve the salmon warm.

If the weather is dry: Serve the salmon chilled on a nest of crisp greens, with lemon wedges for drizzling.

Preheat the oven to 400°F.

Set the fillet skin side down on a large piece of parchment paper or foil. Sprinkle on the jalapeños, garlic, lime, and salt, then cover all with the lemon slices. Seal the parchment or foil by folding it together, then set the package in a baking pan and bake until the salmon is cooked through, 15 to 20 minutes. Serve warm, at room temperature, or slightly chilled for a lunch or dinner entrée.

MAKES 4 SERVINGS; 205 CALORIES PER SERVING; 9 GRAMS OF FAT; 38 PERCENT OF CALORIES FROM FAT.

VARIATION:

For a quick and cooler cooking method, microwave the salmon by preparing it in the parchment paper, and then setting the package on a large dinner plate. Microwave on full power for 4 to 5 minutes, then let the fish relax, before unwrapping, for about 3 minutes more.

grilled salmon with mustard and fennel

If the weather is damp:
Serve a side dish of
steamed new potatoes
tossed with spicy salsa.

If the weather is dry: Serve
a side dish of steamed
sugar snap peas tossed
with sautéed mushrooms
and fresh lemon juice.

Try this dish after a spring day has left you frazzled—mustard and fennel are what herbalists call carminatives, substances that help soothe stressed digestion.

12 ounces salmon fillet   **1 tablespoon fennel seeds**
2 tablespoons prepared mustard

Prepare the grill or preheat the broiler.

Spread the salmon flesh with the mustard, then sprinkle on the fennel seeds. Grill or broil the salmon about 4 inches from the heat source until just cooked through, about 4 minutes on each side. Serve warm or at room temperature for a brunch, lunch, or dinner entrée.

MAKES 4 SERVINGS; 200 CALORIES PER SERVING; 9 GRAMS OF FAT; 40 PERCENT OF CALORIES FROM FAT.

salmon with fresh dill

If the weather is damp:
Serve the salmon warm
with a side dish of curry-
scented, steamed new
potatoes.

If the weather is dry: Serve
the salmon chilled with a
side dish of chilled,
steamed asparagus
(see pages 118–125).

With the taste of lemon and celery, dillweed perfumes the salmon without over-powering the flavor. In addition, this feathery springtime herb contains volatile oils that help soothe digestive distress.

2 teaspoons prepared mustard   **1 tablespoon minced fresh dillweed**
2 tablespoons rice vinegar   **12 ounces salmon fillet**

Prepare the grill or preheat the broiler.

In a small bowl, combine the mustard, vinegar, and dill. Spread the salmon flesh with the mixture, then grill or broil, about 4 inches from the heat source, until the salmon is just cooked, about 4 minutes on each side. Serve warm, at room temperature, or very slightly chilled for a brunch, lunch, or dinner entrée.

MAKES 4 SERVINGS; 200 CALORIES PER SERVING; 9 GRAMS OF FAT; 40 PERCENT OF CALORIES FROM FAT.

salmon with spring herb paste

For those who are retaining water this spring, the herbs in this fragrant dish are strong enough to eliminate the need for salt.

2 cloves garlic

1 tablespoon chopped fresh tarragon

1 tablespoon chopped fresh parsley

1 tablespoon chopped fresh thyme

¼ cup lemon juice

12 ounces salmon fillet

Prepare the grill or preheat the broiler.

In a food processor or blender, combine the garlic, tarragon, parsley, thyme, and lemon juice and process until smooth. Spread the paste on the salmon flesh and grill or broil about 4 inches from the heat source until the fillet is just cooked through, about 4 minutes on each side. Serve warm, at room temperature, or slightly chilled for a brunch, lunch, or dinner entrée.

MAKES 4 SERVINGS; 200 CALORIES PER SERVING; 9 GRAMS OF FAT; 40 PERCENT OF CALORIES FROM FAT.

If the weather is damp: Serve the salmon warm, sprinkled liberally with freshly ground black pepper.

If the weather is dry: Serve the salmon slightly chilled, drizzled with fresh lemon juice.

spicy salmon salad

If the weather is damp:
Serve with hot ginger tea.

If the weather is dry: Serve
with chilled peppermint or
sage tea.

This zippy dish provides the perfect warmth for a chilly or drizzly spring day. The chili powder adds warmth to the body, and the arugula contributes a peppery glow.

2 tablespoons lemon juice

1 teaspoon good-quality chili powder, or to taste

Splash of hot pepper sauce, or to taste

2 scallions, minced

1 clove garlic, minced

Pinch of sea salt

½ cup plain nonfat yogurt or soy yogurt

12 ounces salmon fillet, cooked, broken into bite-sized pieces

2 cups spring greens, such as arugula or cress

In a medium bowl, combine the lemon juice, chili powder, hot pepper sauce, scallions, garlic, salt, and yogurt. Gently fold in the salmon and toss until all of the pieces are coated with the dressing. Arrange the greens on 4 plates and scoop on the salmon mixture. Serve as a brunch, lunch, or dinner entrée.

MAKES 4 SERVINGS; 216 CALORIES PER SERVING; 9 GRAMS OF FAT; 33 PERCENT OF CALORIES FROM FAT.

IDEAS FOR LIGHT SPRING MENUS

Spring cooking is easy, because the season's offerings—greens, peas, and asparagus, for instance—are virtually effortless to prepare. These menus illustrate the point, and I hope they will inspire you to devise your own.

Mellow Spring Lunch: The magnesium in the mustard greens acts as a soothing spring tonic. Magnesium's absence from the diet is associated with irritability and depression. The mints in the tea contain aromatic oils that act as a calming carminative to stressed digestion.

* Mixed Mint Tea (page 82)
* Mustard Greens Salad, Vietnamese Style (page 96)
* Fresh Strawberry Sherbet (page 134)

Spring Cleaning Dinner: Many of the ingredients in this menu, such as catnip, asparagus, and the spring greens, act as gentle diuretics to help banish seasonal bloat.

* Soothing Catnip Tonic (page 84)
* Penne with Garlic-Simmered Asparagus (page 121)
* Spring Greens with Fresh Herb Dressing (page 95)
* (Fresh strawberries sprinkled with) Strawberry Vinegar (page 130)

Best of the Season: This brunch, lunch, or dinner feast combines such wonderful spring offerings as salmon, watercress, asparagus, and strawberries.

* Bay-Steamed Asparagus (page 120)
* Grilled Salmon with Mustard and Fennel (page 138)
* Watercress Salad with Artichokes and Balsamic Vinaigrette (page 94)
* Lemon Cake with Fresh Strawberries (page 133)

Make-Your-Own Spring Meal: Make these condiments ahead and they'll be ready to enhance your favorite spring foods.

* Fresh Spinach Sauce with Chives (page 89). Serve in a pool on a plate with grilled or poached and chilled salmon atop; toss with cooked linguine; use as the dressing for a lentil or white bean salad; drizzle atop steamed asparagus.

* Dandelion Vinegar (page 97). Toss with chopped Vidalia onions, a splash of olive oil, and freshly ground pepper for an instant relish; combine with an equal part of prepared mustard and use as a marinade for grilled salmon; toss with watercress and fresh chopped tomato.

* Fresh Strawberry Jam (page 131). Spread on pancakes or waffles; mix with an equal part of nonfat vanilla yogurt and use as a dip for fresh fruit slices; spread on an oatmeal cookie, then top with a second cookie.

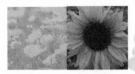

gateway
from spring
to summer

a s dewy spring ripens into the intense heat of summer, my cats shed. It's a messy time, requiring extra grooming and vacuuming. I like it, because as my cats cast off their winter coats to be more comfortable, it's a message for me to do the same. I trade boots and leggings for bare legs and painted toenails; thick jackets and trousers for light, strappy dresses.

It is then that I, along with millions of others, indulge the urge to grow things, luring tiny shoots up through the newly warmed earth, as symbols of renewal and growth. I recommend growing herbs, because their aromas, tastes, and therapeutic qualities are irresistible. Many varieties will grow in a pot on a windowsill that gets at least six hours of sun a day. If needed, you can augment the light with a halogen desk lamp with the light source about three feet away from the leaves of the plant and left on up to twelve hours a day. Try rosemary, thyme, tarragon, chives, oregano, and basil. Snip the leaves into green salads or sprinkle them atop vegetable, rice, and pasta dishes to taste.

If you have garden space, you can grow herbs in a raised bed. To do so, design one or more areas that fit your space, in a square, triangle, or rectangle. Size each bed so you can reach all the plants inside without having to step in. Then press two-by-eight-inch wooden boards, in lengths that match your design, into the first couple of inches of soil, and nail them together. Fill in the bed with a mixture of two parts potting soil, two parts peat, one part sand, and one part composted cow manure.

Select herbs for planting that you like to use dried in cooking and teas. Some herbs, such as mustard greens and sorrel, can be planted as soon as the soil is no longer frozen. More delicate herbs, like basil, should be planted after Mother's Day to ensure happy growing. Herbs such as rosemary and sage, which come back each year, grow well together because sage helps keep rosemary from developing powdery mildew. Add peppermint (in a bottomless pot to keep its lateral roots from spreading), chives, petunias, and marigolds along the edges to deter aphids, bunnies, and other pests, and you have a fragrant herb garden. Water it when the soil is dry, and discard dead leaves and twigs regularly to help discourage infestations.

More Activities to Evoke a Summery Mood: Buy a gorgeous pair of sandals. Get a pedicure. Change to a lighter, more refreshing fragrance. Purchase a cool new pair of sunglasses. Walk to work. Eat more fresh, raw vegetables and fruits. Drink more water. Send jokes by e-mail. Wear a great straw hat. Be open to new ideas.

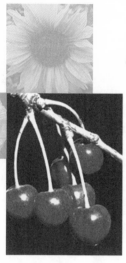

summer:
the season
of growth

may, june, july

BEST TIME OF YEAR FOR:

* *Taking action on the ideas you formulated in the spring*

* *Being energetic; exercising your mind and body*

* *Learning something new*

Country music drifts from a portable radio as I sit in the semi-shaded entrance of a small trading post near Two Grey Hills, Arizona, one mid-July noon. A Navajo medicine man tells me, "Heat from the sun is what gives all life energy, and like the corn that grows, summer gives strength and vitality to people, too."

"If that's true," I inquired, "then why am I sometimes so fatigued in summer?"

If you work with the sun it will make you strong, he explained. Work against it, and it will weaken you. Copy the lizards, who rest as the day gets hotter. Do more strenuous physical exercise in the cooler morning or evening, slowing your body down and refreshing it during the hotter midday. I saw his point, recalling how the previous day my lack of respect for desert heat sent me hiking up Tapatio Cliffs around noon. Upon feeling faint and unable to breathe normally, I stopped in the shade to drink what water I had, then slowly made my way down the hill. I had quickly learned the lesson of working with the summer sun, planning subsequent and more energizing hikes at dawn and dusk.

Similarly, an African doctor in Zimbabwe told me that as temperatures soar and the ambient, or outside, temperature creeps up to be comparable to our body temperature, breathing and other simple

THE MONTH OF MAY
The fifth month was named for the Roman earth goddess, Maia, in hopes that she would provide direction and strength to all life on earth. May is a time to unfold and bloom.

149

INTERESTING DATES IN MAY

May 1—Beltane, the ancient Celtic festival announcing the bright half of the year, where participants celebrated by dancing, singing, and kindling flames anew.

May 5—Feast of Banners in Japan, a celebration honoring the active, warm part of the year, during which all that is masculine and fiery is celebrated.

May 21 (approximate)—The sun enters the zodiac sign of Gemini—the Twins—symbolizing communication and intellectual pursuits.

body functions become difficult. But by slowing down during the hot midday, we rest and store energy. Our bodies, he said, want us to be like big African cats hanging in a tree until the temperature cools down and we can comfortably be more physically active. The same principle works in New York City, where sweltering days are relatively quiet and some offices close early. But as the sun goes down, the streets come alive with people, animated and hungry, perhaps for the first time all day.

Chinese healers, too, believe that summer sun vitalizes the mind and body, and that both should be exercised appropriately to prevent imbalances. Outdoor recreation is critical or "heat disharmonies" could occur, including headaches, rashes, fatigue, irritability, body aches, and respiratory complaints. A Western scientist might explain this by noting how basking in the sun, even for a mere fifteen minutes very early in the morning, activates the body's ability to manufacture vitamin D, a nutrient that is essential for calcium absorption. Without vitamin D and calcium, the aforementioned health conditions may arise, as well as high blood pressure, osteoporosis, and colon cancer.

It is quite possible to grow and even flourish in the summer season by heeding how your mind and body respond to the immediate environment. Try exercising, playing, and working hard both mentally and physically, but if the fire's too hot, wait until later. Taking that to the extreme, the Centers for Disease Control and Prevention, studying the 1995 heat wave that killed over seven hundred people in Chicago, advise that air conditioning, especially midday, can help prevent illness and even death. You may also wish to try the following refreshing tips and recipes.

first aid kit for summer

You probably have some of these useful items on hand right now, such as honey and vinegar. If not, try to keep a few around, especially those you know you'll need.

Cool Your Skin—For relief from sunburn, run a warm (not hot) bath. While the water is flowing, tie an herb bag or a cheesecloth bag of dried chamomile tea flowers to the faucet, letting the water filter through it. To the water itself add a cup of rolled oats, or a packet of colloidal oatmeal (easily dispersed), available at pharmacies. Soak in the tub for about twenty minutes. Both the oats and chamomile contain compounds that calm inflamed skin. As an alternative, add half a cup of cider vinegar to the warm bathwater and soak for twenty minutes. The vinegar helps heal skin by correcting the skin's pH. The oat and vinegar baths will also temporarily abate discomfort from poison ivy.

To make your own cooling skin elixir, combine a quarter cup of aloe vera gel with five drops of essential oil of lavender, and apply three times a day to the affected area. Aloe is what experts call an "external demulcent," a substance that soothes skin and helps it heal. Lavender has vulnerary properties, which means it, too, helps skin mend.

For more after-bath renewal, make your own herbal body powder by combining half a cup of cornstarch with two tablespoons of ground, dried lavender flowers.

As a take-along cooler, carry a small spray bottle filled with spring water to mist your face, or any part of you that needs to be revived. For extra refreshment, you may also wish to add about fifteen drops of essential oil of lavender (to each half cup of water) and spray as needed—in the subway, in your car in heavy traffic, at the office, at a picnic, at a smoky cocktail party.

Cool Rashes, Cuts, Scratches, Bites, and Blisters—Dot pure honey on washed cuts and scratches. Its comforting, antibacterial action will fortify the healing process. For enhanced healing action you may also wish to empty a capsule of powdered echinacea herb into a tablespoon of honey before applying. This potion takes the sting out of bug bites. Half a teaspoon of tincture of yarrow, comfrey, or calendula, available at herb shops and natural food stores, can also be added to a tablespoon of honey to amplify treatment for cuts, scratches, and bites. The calendula combination will help calm itchy rashes, including poison ivy. For blisters, wash the area well before covering with a fresh sage leaf or plantain (Plantago) leaf, changing the green dressing every two hours.

THE MONTH OF JUNE
The sixth month was named for Juno, Roman goddess and Queen of Heaven, who was believed to cast light upon the creative powers of those on earth below.

INTERESTING DATES IN JUNE
June 16—Night of the Drop in Egypt, when the waters of the river Nile reach their lowest point, baring a cache of rich bottom soil and illustrating that the time is right for growth, both in the garden and elsewhere. *June 21 (approximate)—Summer Solstice*, marking the longest day of the year. Some herbalists say this is the best day to harvest herbs for healing teas. This is also the day the sun enters the zodiac sign of Cancer the Crab, a symbol of intuition and hospitality.

THE MONTH OF JULY

THE MONTH OF JULY
The seventh month was named for the Roman general Julius Caesar. In China, this month is represented by a dragon for strength, and the lotus flower for longevity.

INTERESTING DATES IN JULY
July 20—Binding of the Wreaths in Lithuania, where lovers wind flowers into wreaths to symbolize the weaving together of their lives. *July 23* (approximate)—The sun enters the zodiac sign of Leo, symbolizing generosity and energy. In ancient Gaul this day was called *Elembiuos*, or "claim time," during which any unmet obligations were fulfilled.

Cool Your Aches and Pains—If a weekend of activity has left your muscles sore, relax them in a warm Epsom salts bath. Dissolve one to two cups of the soothing salts in the running water and soak for about twenty minutes.

Cool the Insects—To make your own insect repellent, in a spray bottle combine one cup of liquid witch hazel (available at pharmacies and supermarkets), one tablespoon of cider vinegar, and two 4-inch sprigs of fresh rosemary. Spray your skin and the area around you, repeating every twenty minutes. Make the mixture ahead so it will be ready when you need it; it keeps for about two weeks. Also note that since many biting and stinging insects are attracted to sweets, peel and eat that banana indoors.

cooling summer beverages

Lack of sufficient liquids to keep the body hydrated is a major cause of summer fatigue and irritability. On a commonsense level this seems obvious, but scientists have validated the notion in a number of alertness tests, the results of which indicate that people perform better mentally and physically when they are hydrated. Thirst, of course, is one way to tell if you need a drink, but since dehydration may occur on more subtle bodily levels—such as muddled thinking and sluggishness—it's a good idea to drink eight 8-ounce glasses of water a day, or try these rejuvenating summer beverages.

refreshing moon teas

If the weather is damp: Add a small cinnamon stick to the brew before steeping overnight.

If the weather is dry: Add a slice of fresh lemon to the brew before steeping overnight. Or add a slice of dried licorice root, available at natural food stores and Asian markets.

This simple technique is one I learned in Egypt. It's technically called a "cold infusion" because it uses room temperature water rather than boiling water. Moon tea seems an apt name, since the brew is steeped overnight in lunar light. Making these vitalizing and delightful teas is one of the nicest things you can do for yourself this summer.

2 handfuls fresh herbs
   (about 1 cup not packed)

1 quart water, at room temperature

Combine the herbs and water in a glass container and let the mixture infuse overnight. In the morning discard the herbs and enjoy the brew throughout the day. You can also pour the tea into a container to take to work.

MAKES FOUR 1–CUP SERVINGS; 3 TO 5 CALORIES PER SERVING; NO ADDED FAT.

IDEAS FOR MOON TEA COMBINATIONS:
Digestive Tonics—Equal parts tarragon and mint.
   Equal parts mint, oregano, and bee balm; plus a 2-inch ribbon of lemon peel.
Sinus Openers—Equal parts hyssop and sage.
   Equal parts sage and rosemary (for sinus headache).
Anxiety Soother—Equal parts basil and lemon balm.

fresh fruit tea

A Thai chef taught me to make this tea. It's a guaranteed refresher, even in a steamy Bangkok kitchen.

2 strawberries, sliced
1 orange segment, chopped
2 sprigs fresh mint

2 teaspoons black tea leaves, or herb
   tea of your choice
2 cups just-boiled water

Combine all of the ingredients, and steep, covered, for about 2 minutes. Discard the fruit and tea leaves, and sip.

MAKES TWO 1–CUP SERVINGS; 5 CALORIES PER SERVING; NO ADDED FAT.

If the weather is damp: Sip the tea warm or hot.

If the weather is dry: Sip the tea slightly chilled.

calm mind tea

If a hot day has aggravated your mood, try this soothing herbal combination.

½ teaspoon dried chamomile flowers
½ teaspoon dried linden flowers

1 teaspoon dried lavender flowers
1 cup just-boiled water

Combine all of the ingredients and steep, covered, for 4 minutes. Strain and sip.

MAKES ONE SERVING; 3 CALORIES PER SERVING; NO ADDED FAT.

If the weather is damp: Add a pinch of rosemary to the tea before steeping; sip warm.

If the weather is dry: Swirl in honey to taste, and sip slightly chilled.

wonder woman tea

If the weather is damp: Double the gingerroot and sip the tea warm.

If the weather is dry: Add a slice of lemon to the steeping tea and sip slightly chilled.

Try this pleasant potpourri to help banish bloat and balance hormones.

1 teaspoon dried mint

1 teaspoon dried sage

1 teaspoon dried lemon balm

1 slice fresh gingerroot

1 cup just–boiled water

1 cup just–boiled orange juice

Combine all the ingredients and steep, covered, for 5 minutes.

MAKES TWO 1–CUP SERVINGS; 53 CALORIES PER SERVING; NO ADDED FAT.

egyptian cooler

If the weather is damp: Sip the tea warm.

If the weather is dry: Sip the tea chilled.

This floral beverage is based on hibiscus, which herbalists deem a "refrigerant" to the body. Hibiscus tea is frequently sipped in such blistering locales as Cairo and Khartoum—a testament to its refreshing nature.

2 teaspoons dried hibiscus flowers

1 teaspoon dried mint

2 cups just–boiled water

Steep the hibiscus and mint in the water, covered, for 4 minutes. Then strain and sip.

MAKES TWO 1–CUP SERVINGS; 3 CALORIES PER SERVING; NO ADDED FAT.

olympic orangeade

This was created for a caterer friend who designed menus for the 1996 Olympics in Atlanta, Georgia. The wait staff guzzled it during lunch rush to keep them hydrated and energized while serving 4,000 meals.

If the weather is damp: Stir in a pinch of ground ginger before drinking.

If the weather is dry: Garnish with a sprig of fresh mint.

¾ **cup chilled seltzer water**   ¼ **cup orange juice**

Combine the water and juice and sip.

MAKES ONE SERVING; 26 CALORIES PER SERVING.

gingered lemonade

Prepare the syrup ahead and you'll have an enlivening lemonade anytime you need a boost.

If the weather is damp: Double the amount of gingerroot.

If the weather is dry: Stir the syrup into a cup of chilled peppermint tea.

⅓ **cup honey**   **Juice of 8 lemons**
5 slices fresh gingerroot

In a small saucepan, combine the honey and gingerroot and heat on low until warmed and fragrant, about 5 minutes. Discard the gingerroot and stir in the lemon juice. To use, stir 4 tablespoons of syrup into a cup of plain or seltzer water and enjoy. The syrup will keep, jarred and refrigerated, for about a month. You can also freeze the syrup in ice cube trays and defrost as needed (1 cube equals 2 tablespoons).

MAKES ABOUT 1½ CUPS OF SYRUP, OR SIX ¼-CUP SERVINGS; 58 CALORIES PER SERVING; NO ADDED FAT.

yellow tomato juice

If the weather is damp: Add 2 whole cloves to the spice bag before boiling.

If the weather is dry: Serve the juice slightly chilled, garnished with fresh lemon wedges for squeezing.

A refreshing and hydrating repast, the fennel helps to soothe intestinal-affected summer stress.

2 pounds yellow tomatoes, stemmed, cored, and chopped

1 stick cinnamon

½ teaspoon fennel seeds

1 teaspoon honey

Set the tomatoes in a large saucepan. Tie the cinnamon and fennel seeds together in a piece of cheesecloth or in a spice bag and add to the tomatoes. Stir in the honey. Bring the mixture to a boil, then reduce the heat and simmer gently until fragrant, about 45 minutes, stirring frequently. Remove the spice bag and press the mixture through a food mill or sieve. Serve at room temperature or slightly chilled.

MAKES 1 QUART, OR FOUR 1-CUP SERVINGS; 62 CALORIES PER SERVING; NO ADDED FAT.

spicy tomato juice

If the weather is damp: Stir in a splash of Worcestershire sauce before serving.

If the weather is dry: Stir in a splash of lemon juice before serving.

Rich in potassium, this savory reviver can help to contain high blood pressure levels.

3 pounds ripe red tomatoes

2 pounds ripe plum tomatoes

½ cup chopped onion

2 cloves garlic, sliced

½ celery stalk, chopped, including leaves

2 fresh chile peppers, cored, seeded, and chopped

1 bay leaf

2 sprigs parsley

2 tablespoons lemon juice

1 tablespoon honey

In a large soup pot, combine all of the ingredients and bring to a boil. Reduce the heat and simmer, stirring occasionally, until the vegetables are soft, about 45 minutes. Strain through a sieve or food mill. Serve at room temperature or very slightly chilled.

MAKES FIVE 1-CUP SERVINGS; 121 CALORIES PER SERVING; NO ADDED FAT.

apricot nectar

A good source of immune-enhancing beta carotene, this luscious drink can help avert summer respiratory complaints.

4 cups pitted, sliced ripe apricots   **1 cup hot orange juice**

In a large soup pot, combine the apricots and orange juice and bring to a boil. Reduce the heat and simmer gently until the fruit is very soft, about 45 minutes. Press through a sieve or food mill. To make a beverage of the thick nectar, combine ¼ cup of the nectar with ¾ cup of water, or to taste. Since the nectar is thick, you may also wish to use it undiluted as a dessert sauce for fresh fruit or sorbet.

MAKES 4 CUPS OF NECTAR, OR SIXTEEN ¼-CUP SERVINGS; 57 CALORIES PER SERVING; NO ADDED FAT.

If the weather is damp: Swirl in a pinch of dried gingerroot when making the nectar into a beverage.

If the weather is dry: Garnish with lemon wedges for squeezing.

cooling
summer foods

Chinese healers hold that the body expands in the summer heat, in the same way that a hot compress "expands" or relaxes a contracted muscle. Your shoes may fit a bit more tightly in summer months, and finger rings may be slightly snug. The Chinese feel that this expansion is a cooling and hydrating response to hot weather and advise eating foods that facilitate the effect. Crisp, succulent vegetables such as cucumber, corn, eggplant, tomato, and zucchini are recommended, as are such juicy, cooling fruits as plums, peaches, cherries, mangoes, papayas, and nectarines. Raw food and quick, light styles of cooking such as steaming and grilling are favored to help keep the body comfortable. If baking in a hot oven is required, as may be the case with such foods as eggplant and zucchini, do so in the cooler early or late times of the day.

corn
the heartthrob

Twenty-five summers ago, a handsome young man began to acquaint me, a city dweller, with the various charms of nature. One such delight was a fresh, sweet, baby ear of corn, plucked right from the stalk, peeled, and savored cob and all. The gift of a little ear of corn touched my heart, only adding to the attractiveness of my young man. I married him six months later.

Perhaps it is no coincidence that Chinese and Japanese healers hold that summer corn is a tonic for the heart, and eating it vitalizes and energizes the body. But the Asians aren't alone. In southern Mexico, the Tarahumara Indians eat a diet consisting almost exclusively of corn and beans and suffer virtually no heart disease. Western scientists add that corn contains stress-soothing B vitamins, an additional plus for heart health. Corn is also high in folate, the lack of which may cause summer headaches, indigestion, anxiety, and fatigue. Additionally, corn contains about 85 calories per ear, and one ear yields half a cup of kernels. Each half cup of kernels contains one gram of fat, or 11 percent of calories from fat—more good news for the heart.

gardening and harvesting hints for corn

During the last month of growth, corn can take in a third to a half inch of water a day to accommodate plumping kernels. Be sure to water during drought and during periods of low humidity, or you could lose half your harvest in a mere four days.

Sweet corn is tastiest when picked early in the morning when sugar levels in the kernels are highest. To check for ripeness, press a fingernail into a kernel. If milk spurts right out, the ear is ready to be picked. If clear liquid runs out when a kernel is pressed, the ear is not yet ripe; if the kernel is dry and contains no milk, the ear is past its prime. In some varieties, corn silk or tassels that are dried and brown indicate that the ear is ripe. To double-check, the top of the cob should feel rounded rather than pointed.

* quick cooking tips for corn

To cook corn, shuck and steam the ears until tender; start checking at twelve minutes.

To remove the kernels easily from an ear of corn, hold a shucked cob vertically. Starting at the top, run a horizontally held paring knife down to the bottom, slicing off the kernels as you go. Add half a cup of lightly blanched kernels to a mixed green salad for four, the dough for one loaf of bread, or the batter for pancakes to serve four.

fresh corn salad with tomato vinaigrette

Corn kernels, celery, summer greens, and tomato all cool and rejuvenate the body. In addition, thyme and basil contain aromatic properties that may help lift a sluggish summer mood.

2 cups cooked brown rice
1 cup cooked corn kernels
1/3 cup minced celery
1 shallot, minced
1/2 cup chopped, peeled tomato (page 170)
1 tablespoon lemon juice
1 tablespoon balsamic vinegar
1 teaspoon minced fresh basil, or 1/2 teaspoon dried

1 teaspoon minced fresh thyme, or 1/2 teaspoon dried
1/2 teaspoon Dijon–style mustard
Sea salt and freshly ground pepper to taste
Romaine lettuce leaves for serving

If the weather is damp: Use cooked basmati or other white rice instead of brown rice.

If the weather is dry: Omit the romaine and serve with a crisp green salad on the side.

In a medium bowl, combine the rice, corn, celery, and shallot.

In a blender or food processor, combine the tomato, lemon juice, vinegar, basil, thyme, mustard, salt, and pepper, processing on high until well combined, about 25 seconds. Pour the dressing over the salad and toss well, about 30 times, to coat. Serve at room temperature or very slightly chilled on the romaine leaves for a lunch or dinner entrée.

MAKES 4 SERVINGS; 175 CALORIES PER SERVING; 1 GRAM OF FAT; 5 PERCENT OF CALORIES FROM FAT.

fresh corn crepes

If the weather is damp: Fill the crepes with Pâté of Eggplant, Leek, and Tomato (page 180).

If the weather is dry: Fill the crepes with Herb-Scented Grilled Tomatoes (page 171).

This recipe features corn milk, a cooling, nourishing pale yellow cream made from pureed corn. Stir it into sauces and soups as a low-fat thickener, or use it as a succulent substitute for cream in baking. To make corn milk, simply puree corn kernels in a blender or food processor. One ½ cup of kernels, about the amount from 1 large ear, will yield about ⅓ cup of corn milk.

¼ cup cornmeal

¼ cup unbleached flour

¼ teaspoon ground turmeric

1 egg, 2 egg whites, or ¼ cup commercial egg substitute

½ cup corn milk

½ cup skim or nonfat soy milk

1 tablespoon minced fresh chives

2 teaspoons canola oil

In a medium bowl, combine the cornmeal, flour, and turmeric.

In another medium bowl, combine the egg, egg white, or egg substitute; the corn milk; milk; and chives. Pour the liquid mixture into the cornmeal mixture and stir well to combine. Heat a nonstick crepe pan on high and brush with some oil. Add about 2 tablespoons of batter to the pan, swirling until the batter forms a round crepe. Sizzle until the crepe is burnished with reddish brown, about 2 minutes on each side. Repeat with the remaining batter.

MAKES 16 CREPES (4 ENTRÉE OR 8 SIDE OR APPETIZER SERVINGS); 110 CALORIES PER ENTRÉE SERVING USING EGG WHITES; 2.75 GRAMS OF FAT; 22 PERCENT OF CALORIES FROM FAT.

scallion-studded corn strudel

Corn is a good source of folate, a nutrient that may help prevent summer fatigue. This is especially true for those taking such medications as aspirin, birth control pills, and antacids, as these drugs may deplete the body's store of folate.

1 cup nonfat ricotta cheese or creamy nonfat soy cheese

1½ cups cooked corn kernels

1 cup cooked chopped mustard greens or kale

2 scallions, minced

1 egg, 2 egg whites, or ¼ cup commercial egg substitute

2 tablespoons grated Parmesan cheese or soy Parmesan

6 phyllo dough sheets

2 tablespoons butter or ghee, melted (available at specialty food stores and Indian markets)

⅓ cup whole wheat bread crumbs

If the weather is damp: Add 1 or 2 minced cloves of garlic when you add the scallions.

If the weather is dry: Serve with an accompaniment of juicy tomato wedges.

Preheat the oven to 375°F. Coat a baking sheet with nonstick spray.

In a large bowl, combine the ricotta; corn; mustard greens or kale; scallions; egg, egg whites, or egg substitute; and Parmesan.

Set 2 phyllo sheets on waxed paper. Using a pastry brush, paint the sheets lightly with the butter or ghee, then sprinkle with half of the bread crumbs. Add 2 more sheets, paint, and sprinkle with the remaining crumbs. Add the last 2 phyllo sheets and brush with butter. With the long end of the dough parallel to the edge of your work surface, spread the corn mixture over the dough, leaving an inch on all sides. Using the waxed paper for help, fold the sides of the dough over the mixture so that they cover ½ inch on each side. Brush the edges lightly with water so they don't unfold. With the help of the waxed paper, roll the dough away from you onto the prepared baking sheet. Bake the strudel until lightly browned, about 30 minutes. Serve warm or at room temperature as a brunch, lunch, or dinner entrée.

MAKES 4 SERVINGS; 244 CALORIES PER SERVING; 7 GRAMS OF FAT; 27 PERCENT OF CALORIES FROM FAT.

roasted sweet corn soup with fresh thyme

*If the weather is damp:
Substitute cayenne for the
black pepper.*

—

*If the weather is dry:
Garnish with chopped fresh
tomatoes instead of the
red bell pepper.*

Roasting the ears intensifies their depth of flavor and sweetness without the addition of energy-robbing fats.

4 ears of fresh corn

1 tablespoon unsalted butter or
   olive oil

2 shallots, minced

1 bay leaf

1 tablespoon minced fresh thyme,
   or 1½ teaspoons dried

2 cups low-fat soy, skim, or
   whole milk

Pinch of sea salt

Freshly ground black pepper
   to taste

Red bell pepper slivers for garnish

Minced fresh chives for garnish

To roast the ears, soak them, husk and all, in water to cover for 1 hour. Prepare a grill and arrange the ears on a rack about 4 inches from the heat source. Cover loosely with foil and let the ears roast until they're fragrant and tender, 20 to 25 minutes, turning occasionally. Let the ears cool before shucking and removing the kernels from the cobs. Alternatively, you can shuck the ears first, wrap each in foil, and roast them as directed.

Heat a large sauté pan on medium-high and melt the butter. If you're using olive oil, preheat the pan to avoid sticking. Add the shallots, bay leaf, and thyme, sautéing until the shallots are fragrant and wilted, 4 to 5 minutes.

Discarding the bay leaf, scrape the shallots and thyme into a food processor, along with the corn and 1/2 cup of the milk. Process until the mixture is very smooth.

Pour the mixture into a large saucepan and add the remaining milk. Heat gently on low until warm, about 5 minutes, but don't boil or you'll ruin the texture. Stir in the salt and pepper and serve warm garnished with the red pepper slivers and chives as a lunch entrée, or dinner appetizer.

MAKES 4 SERVINGS; 220 CALORIES PER SERVING; 5.5 GRAMS OF FAT; 23 PERCENT OF CALORIES FROM FAT.

grilled black bean burgers with corn

Since corn is a good source of nerve-soothing B vitamins, this dish is a tonic for summer stresses.

1 teaspoon olive oil	½ cup cooked brown rice
½ cup minced onion	1½ cups cooked black beans
5 whole scallions, minced	1 to 2 cups whole wheat bread
1 cup corn kernels	crumbs
¼ cup good-quality commercial	
tomato salsa	

Heat a medium sauté pan on medium-high heat, then add the oil. Toss in the onion and scallions and sauté until they're lightly browned, 4 to 5 minutes. Stir in the corn and salsa and heat through.

Scoop the corn mixture, rice, beans, and 1 cup of the crumbs into a food processor and blend well. Transfer to a large bowl and check the texture by trying to make a burger. If the mixture doesn't hold together, stir in more bread crumbs.

Prepare the grill or preheat the broiler. Divide the mixture into 8 pieces, shaping each into a firm burger. Arrange the burgers on a fine-mesh grill plate or on a pizza pan, and grill or broil 4 inches from the heat source until lightly browned, about 5 minutes on each side. Serve for a lunch or dinner entrée.

MAKES 8 BURGERS; 165 CALORIES PER BURGER; 1.3 GRAMS OF FAT; 8 PERCENT OF CALORIES FROM FAT.

If the weather is damp: Serve on toasted whole wheat buns with mustard and sliced purple onion.

If the weather is dry: Serve on a bed of curly red lettuce, topped with Herb-Scented Grilled Tomatoes (page 171) or extra tomato salsa.

savory corn cake with tomato-basil sauce

If the weather is damp: Add 1 minced jalapeño pepper with the tomatoes when cooking the sauce.

If the weather is dry: Serve fresh, juicy fruits, such as plums and mangoes, for dessert.

In steamy Brazil, molded polenta, such as these corn cakes, is called *pirão* and is served on sultry evenings to cool and soothe the strains of the day.

2 cups cold plus 2 cups hot
    vegetable stock or water
1 cup cornmeal
½ cup fresh corn kernels
2 pinches of sea salt
1 tablespoon olive oil

2 cloves garlic, minced
1½ pounds tomatoes, seeded and
    chopped
1 teaspoon balsamic vinegar
¼ cup fresh basil, chopped

To make the corn cake, in a medium bowl, combine the cold stock and cornmeal. With the hot stock in a medium saucepan over medium-high heat, stir in the cornmeal mixture, corn kernels, and a pinch of salt. Reduce the heat to medium and continue to stir until the mixture has thickened and starts to release slow bubbles, about 8 minutes.

Lightly oil a 9-inch glass pie plate. Scoop the mixture into the plate and smooth the top. Let the corn cake relax until cool and congealed, about an hour.

To make the sauce, heat a large saucepan on medium-high and pour in the oil. Add the garlic and tomatoes and sauté until the sauce is fragrant and thick, about 10 minutes, stirring in the vinegar, basil, and pinch of salt about a minute before the sauce is done. Serve the corn cake sliced into wedges and drizzled with the sauce, as a lunch or dinner entrée.

MAKES 4 SERVINGS; 190 CALORIES PER SERVING; 4.75 GRAMS OF FAT; 23 PERCENT OF CALORIES FROM FAT.

tomato
pounds of protection

In late July and early August of 1982, I harvested 250 pounds of tomatoes. Needing them to create recipes for two books, I gathered ovals, oblongs, teardrops, currant-sized tomatoes, cherry tomatoes, plums, pears, beefsteaks, heart shapes, and one-pounders that measured six inches across. They were ruby-colored, russet, yellow, white, orange, and striped. And so I became, for that four-week stretch, an authority on picking tomatoes. One tip to encourage a high yield is to harvest daily. Also, pick tomatoes before they become soft by tenderly twisting ripe specimens from the stem; don't pull. If a tomato doesn't come away easily, it's not ripe and shouldn't be harvested. I also noticed that tomato plants bearing fruits that ripened evenly were mulched, a practice that also keeps the fruits clean.

While foraging for my fruits, I learned that in Pennsylvania Dutch folk medicine, a diet high in fresh, unsalted tomatoes is recommended to clear uric acid from the body, thus easing the pain of gout. Nor have tomatoes escaped the eye of modern science, which reveals that they contain a carotene compound called "lycopene" that helps protect against lung cancer and prostate cancer when tomatoes are eaten at least fifteen times a month.

As for protection from summer dehydration, tomatoes are 94 percent water, making them a wonderfully refreshing snack. In addition, an average-sized tomato contains about 30 calories and virtually no fat.

how many tomatoes in a pound?

1 pound = 30 cherry tomatoes
       = 8 plum tomatoes
       = 3 or 4 average salad tomatoes
       = ½ to 1 beefsteak tomato

quick cooking tip for tomatoes

Although the skins are high in digestion-enhancing fiber, you may wish to remove them to avoid bitterness in long-cooking recipes. To do so, immerse tomatoes in boiling water for thirty to sixty seconds, depending on their size. Then plunge them directly into ice water for about ten seconds. The skins will have started to peel away, and you can easily finish the job. Tomatoes, peeled or not, add zest to salsas, salads, sauces, soups, stews, sautés, and casseroles. Or, mince ripe specimens along with garlic and fresh basil and enjoy them on crusty bread instead of butter.

herb-scented grilled tomatoes

Tomatoes, such as the ones in this wonderfully perfumed recipe, contain heart-healthy potassium, which may be depleted from the body during hot summer weather.

16 plum tomatoes (about 2 pounds)
2 tablespoons cider vinegar
1 tablespoon balsamic vinegar
1 teaspoon olive oil

5 fresh basil leaves
2 cloves garlic, minced
1 tablespoon minced fresh thyme, or
  1½ teaspoons dried

Prepare the grill or preheat the broiler. Seed and drain the tomatoes. Then grill or broil them about 5 inches from the heat source for 5 minutes on one side and 2 minutes on the other, until the skins become blistered and slightly charred.

In a large glass baking dish, combine the remaining ingredients.

When the tomatoes have cooled enough to handle, discard the skins and set the tomatoes in a single layer in the marinade, spooning some marinade over each tomato. Cover and let the tomatoes marinate for at least an hour, but they will keep, refrigerated, for about 5 days. Chop and toss with just-cooked pasta, or serve the tomatoes with crusty bread as a lunch entrée or as an appetizer before dinner.

MAKES 4 SERVINGS; 65 CALORIES PER SERVING; 1 GRAM OF FAT; 14 PERCENT OF CALORIES FROM FAT.

If the weather is damp: Add an extra clove of garlic to the marinade, then chop the tomatoes and serve atop crisp French bread as an open-faced sandwich.

If the weather is dry: Chop the tomatoes and toss (with the marinade) with pasta or rice.

tomato salad with red onion and watercress

If the weather is damp: Add a splash of hot pepper sauce to the dressing before whisking.

If the weather is dry: Substitute fresh or dried mint for the basil and oregano.

Moist tomatoes provide a refreshing repast. As a bonus, the purple onion in this dish contains compounds that can help clear summer respiratory complaints.

1 tablespoon cider vinegar

1 tablespoon balsamic vinegar

1 teaspoon minced fresh basil, or ½ teaspoon dried

1 teaspoon minced fresh oregano, or ½ teaspoon dried

1 teaspoon prepared mustard

4 large tomatoes, cored and cut into wedges

1 medium red onion, thinly sliced

¼ cup watercress leaves

In a medium bowl, combine the cider and balsamic vinegars, basil, oregano, and mustard, whisking to combine. Gently stir in the tomatoes, onion, and watercress, cover, and refrigerate for about 2 hours. Toss well before serving slightly chilled for lunch or dinner.

MAKES 4 SERVINGS; 40 CALORIES PER SERVING; NO ADDED FAT.

spicy tomato grill sauce

If the weather is damp: Be generous when adding the red pepper flakes.

If the weather is dry: Paint on moist foods, such as tofu or sea scallops.

The red pepper and celery seed contain aromatic properties that help to soothe summer indigestion.

1 cup finely chopped tomatoes

¼ cup red wine vinegar

1 tablespoon Worcestershire sauce

1 teaspoon crushed red pepper flakes, or to taste

2 cloves garlic, minced

1 teaspoon celery seed

1 bay leaf

Freshly ground black pepper to taste

In a medium saucepan, combine all of the ingredients and bring them to a boil. Reduce the heat, cover loosely, and simmer until the sauce is fragrant, 15 to 20 minutes, stirring frequently. Let the sauce cool slightly before pressing through a strainer. To use, paint on such foods as eggplant, zucchini, tofu, or fish during the last minutes of grilling.

MAKES ABOUT 1 CUP, OR 4 SERVINGS; 37 CALORIES PER SERVING; NO ADDED FAT.

fresh tomato sauce

Summer-ripe tomatoes make this no-cook sauce an easily prepared and rejuvenating repast.

8 small to medium tomatoes, cored, seeded, and chopped

1 clove garlic, finely minced

2 teaspoons balsamic vinegar

2 tablespoons minced fresh basil

Pinch of sea salt

Freshly ground black pepper to taste

In a medium bowl, combine all of the ingredients and let them marinate, at room temperature, for 1 hour before serving atop a pound (to serve 4) of grilled fish or poultry, or tossed with 4 cups of cooked pasta.

MAKES 4 SERVINGS; 55 CALORIES PER SERVING; NO ADDED FAT.

If the weather is damp: Use 2 cloves of garlic, and be generous with the black pepper.

If the weather is dry: Serve with cold poached salmon or with chilled, steamed vegetables.

tomato soup with garlic and dill

If the weather is damp:
Serve the soup warm,
garnished with minced
fresh chives and crisp
croutons.

If the weather is dry: Serve
the soup slightly chilled
with lemon wedges for
squeezing.

Dillweed offers aromatic properties that can help calm hot weather–induced indigestion.

1 tablespoon olive oil

1 medium carrot, finely minced

1 celery stalk, finely minced

1 leek, topped, tailed, and finely minced

1 bay leaf

18 large plum tomatoes, peeled and chopped

2 cloves garlic, peeled and thinly sliced

1 teaspoon minced fresh dillweed

Pinch of sea salt

Freshly ground black pepper to taste

Heat a large soup pot on medium-high, then pour in the olive oil. Add the carrot, celery, leek, and bay leaf. Sauté until they're fragrant and tender, 10 to 15 minutes.

Add the tomatoes (including juices), garlic, dillweed, salt, and pepper and simmer, loosely covered, until the tomatoes have become soft, about 20 minutes. Let the soup cool for about 20 minutes.

Scoop the soup, in batches, into a food processor and process until the soup is almost smooth but is still a bit chunky, about 5 seconds. Serve warm, at room temperature, or slightly chilled for lunch or dinner.

MAKES 4 SERVINGS; 106 CALORIES PER SERVING; 3.5 GRAMS OF FAT; 30 PERCENT OF CALORIES FROM FAT.

tomato sorbet

This refreshing dessert can help cool your digestion and your mood.

6 medium tomatoes, coarsely
  chopped
1 tablespoon lemon juice
½ teaspoon grated lemon zest

⅓ cup honey, or to taste
Pinch of ground cinnamon
Pinch of freshly grated nutmeg

If the weather is damp: Be generous when adding the cinnamon.

If the weather is dry: This is the perfect restorative end to a summer meal.

Puree the tomatoes in a food processor or blender, and press them through a fine sieve to remove and discard the peels and seeds. You'll have about 3 cups of juice.

In an ice cream maker, combine the tomato juice with the remaining ingredients and process according to the manufacturer's instructions.

MAKES 4 LARGE DESSERT SERVINGS; 115 CALORIES PER SERVING; NO ADDED FAT.

eggplant
the stomach soother

Gazing dreamily across the Strait of Malacca to the island of Sumatra, I sat on the beach at Port Dixon, Malaysia, expanding my eggplant horizons. Mr. Lem, a cook, gardener, and Jamu medicine man, was explaining that eggplant comes from India and China, where the original varieties were white ovals; hence the name. Mr. Lem had with him a crock of purple-and-white-swirled eggplant the size of acorns, which he planned to simmer with tomatoes, garlic, and onion, for our lunch. Mr. Lem grew "snake" eggplant—long, slender, curved fruits with a purple hue; yellow ovals; violet-and-white-striped ovals; and deep purple pear-shaped eggplant, similar to yet slightly more petite than the variety familiar to western cooks.

Mr. Lem proclaimed that vegetarians should eat eggplant every day, because it aids in the digestion of a vegetable-based and whole-grain diet. Western medicine might explain this by noting that eggplant contains guar gum, a type of fiber that is soothing to the intestines. In addition, guar gum may help lower blood cholesterol levels by capturing saturated fats in the intestines before these fats enter the bloodstream. Another plus, especially in summer heat, is that half a cup of chopped, cooked eggplant contains virtually no fat and a mere 20 calories.

for excellent eggplant

Whether in the garden or at the market, a vivid green cap and glossy skin indicate ripeness and freshness. Press the eggplant's skin with your finger. If it does not bounce back, the flesh will be moist with small, nonbitter seeds. Since eggplant perishes quickly, harvest or buy only as much as you need, and store it in the refrigerator.

quick cooking tips for eggplant

Although eggplant can be easily grilled and steamed (as the recipes in this section illustrate), microwaving is quick and cool. Peel and chop an eggplant so that you have about two cups of evenly sized pieces. Arrange them in a glass pie dish and sprinkle on about a quarter cup of water. Cover with vented plastic wrap and microwave on full power until the eggplant is tender, about five minutes. Let it relax for about three minutes, then drain. Use the eggplant in marinated vegetable salads, vegetable sautés, sauces, and soups, and as a light and refreshing alternative to meat in such dishes as moussaka and lasagne.

roasted eggplant spread

*If the weather is damp:
Add hot pepper sauce to
taste when pureeing the
spread, and serve on
toasted whole wheat pita
fans.*

*If the weather is dry: Use
as a dip for such cooling
vegetables as cherry
tomatoes, celery sticks,
and cucumber rounds.*

In addition to eggplant's summer-soothing digestive properties, this savory spread contains calcium-rich tahini (sesame butter) that helps fight hot-weather fatigue.

1 medium eggplant
⅓ cup minced fresh parsley
¼ cup lemon juice
¼ cup tahini (sesame butter)

2 cloves garlic, mashed through a
  press
Pinch of sea salt

Preheat the oven to 500°F. and lightly oil a glass pie plate.

Set the whole unpeeled eggplant in the pie plate and bake until the skin is charred and the flesh is soft, about 45 minutes. Alternatively you can halve the eggplant and microwave the halves, cut side down, on waxed paper, on full power until tender, about 15 minutes. This method produces silky flesh, and although the flavor will be unroasted, your kitchen will be cooler.

Scoop the eggplant out of the skin into a food processor or blender and process until smooth, adding the parsley, lemon juice, tahini, garlic, and salt as you go. (Discard the skin.) Let the spread cool, covered and refrigerated, for an hour or so before serving slightly chilled or at room temperature as a spread, dip, or sandwich filling.

MAKES 8 SERVINGS; 75 CALORIES PER SERVING; 3 GRAMS OF FAT; 35 PERCENT OF CALORIES FROM FAT.

summer vegetable soup

Eggplant, tomatoes, celery, basil, and thyme combine to create a fragrant and balancing dish for a hot, tired, overworked mind and body.

1 medium eggplant, peeled and cut into 1-inch chunks

6 medium tomatoes, cored, seeded, and chopped (including juice)

1 red bell pepper, cored, seeded, and chopped

1 onion, chopped

2 celery stalks, sliced

2 cloves garlic, minced

2 cups vegetable stock or water

1 tablespoon minced fresh thyme, or 1½ teaspoons dried

1 tablespoon minced fresh basil, or 1½ teaspoons dried

2 teaspoons olive oil

Pinch of sea salt

If the weather is damp: Swirl in freshly ground pepper before serving warm in shallow bowls with crusty whole-grain baguettes.

If the weather is dry: Serve slightly chilled, garnished with chopped, ripe tomatoes.

In a large soup pot, combine the vegetables, garlic, and stock or water and bring to a boil. Reduce the heat, cover loosely, and simmer, stirring frequently, until the soup is fragrant and the vegetables are very soft, about 25 minutes. Swirl in the thyme, basil, olive oil, and salt, and serve warm, at room temperature, or slightly chilled for lunch or dinner.

MAKES 4 SERVINGS; 90 CALORIES PER SERVING; 2.2 GRAMS OF FAT; 20 PERCENT OF CALORIES FROM FAT.

pâté of eggplant, leek, and tomato

If the weather is damp: Add a minced fresh jalapeño pepper when adding the tomatoes, and serve at room temperature or warmed.

If the weather is dry: Swirl in a squeeze of lemon juice before serving slightly chilled.

A barely detectable hint of golden turmeric gives this thick, aromatic sandwich spread what Ayurvedic healers call a "cooling, soothing" nature.

2 teaspoons olive oil
2 medium eggplant, cubed
¼ cup vegetable stock or water
2 leeks, topped, tailed, and chopped
3 cloves garlic, minced
2 red bell peppers, diced
2 zucchini, cubed

6 medium tomatoes, cored, seeded, and chopped
¼ cup raisins
1 teaspoon minced fresh rosemary, or ½ teaspoon dried
½ teaspoon ground turmeric
Pinch of sea salt

Heat a large sauté pan on medium-high and add the oil. Add the eggplant and stock or water, sautéing until the eggplant has just begun to soften, 4 to 5 minutes. Stir in the remaining ingredients, reduce the heat to medium, and continue to sauté until the pâté is thick and fragrant, 20 to 25 minutes. Serve warm, at room temperature, or very slightly chilled with carrot sticks for dipping; enjoy on sandwiches or as a spread for toasted French bread rounds.

MAKES 4 LARGE SERVINGS; 172 CALORIES PER SERVING; 2.2 GRAMS OF FAT; 10 PERCENT OF CALORIES FROM FAT.

garlicky grilled eggplant

Chinese, Ayurvedic, and Unani (Arabic) healers consider yogurt, of which the marinade in this recipe is composed, to be an antianxiety, cooling food. The addition of mint gives an even more cooling aspect, since the herb contains compounds that, when ingested, activate the cold nerve receptors on the skin.

½ cup plain nonfat yogurt or soy yogurt

3 cloves garlic, minced

2 tablespoons minced fresh mint

1 tablespoon minced fresh oregano

Pinch of sea salt

1 large eggplant, cut into 1½-inch chunks

20 red and yellow cherry tomatoes

If the weather is damp: Liberally add freshly ground black pepper to the marinade, and serve warm.

If the weather is dry: Serve with chilled mint tea.

In a flat glass baking dish, combine the yogurt, garlic, mint, oregano, and salt. Add the eggplant chunks, tossing them in the marinade until they are well coated. Let the eggplant marinate at room temperature for about 20 minutes.

Meanwhile, preheat the broiler or prepare the grill. Thread the eggplant chunks and tomatoes on skewers (reserve the marinade) and grill about 4 inches from the heat source until the eggplant is tender, 2 to 3 minutes on each side. Serve warm or at room temperature as a lunch or dinner entrée, using the reserved marinade as a dipping sauce.

MAKES 4 SERVINGS; 60 CALORIES PER SERVING; NO ADDED FAT.

eggplant with tomato and basil

If the weather is damp:
Serve the eggplant as a
warm sandwich on crusty
bread.

If the weather is dry: Serve
the eggplant at room
temperature or slightly
chilled, with a lively green
salad.

Ayurvedic herbalists say that basil is soothing, cooling, and promotes harmony after a day of stress.

1 large eggplant, peeled and thinly sliced
2 teaspoons olive oil
1 tablespoon freshly grated Parmesan cheese or soy Parmesan

2 tablespoons minced fresh basil
2 ripe tomatoes, sliced
¼ cup grated nonfat mozzarella or soy mozzarella

Preheat the oven to 375°F. Lightly oil a 9-inch glass pie dish.

Steam the eggplant over boiling water until the eggplant is just tender, 7 to 8 minutes. For a cooler method, put the eggplant in a glass pie dish with 1 tablespoon of water, cover, and microwave on full power for about 3 minutes, then let it stand for 2 minutes.

Arrange half the eggplant on the bottom of the pie dish. Sprinkle on half the olive oil, half the Parmesan, and all of the basil. Cover with half of the tomatoes, then start the layering process again with the eggplant, olive oil, and (not all of the) Parmesan, ending with tomatoes and the rest of the Parmesan on top.

Bake uncovered until the eggplant is fragrant and cooked through, about 20 minutes, sprinkling on the mozzarella about halfway through the baking. Alternatively, microwave, covered, on full power for about 8 minutes. Then add the mozzarella and continue to microwave on medium power until the mozzarella is melted, about 2 minutes more. Serve warm or at room temperature as a side dish or as an entrée for brunch, lunch, or dinner.

MAKES 4 SERVINGS; 80 CALORIES PER SERVING; 2.75 GRAMS OF FAT; 27 PERCENT OF CALORIES FROM FAT.

eggplant steaks with silky garlic

After a long, hot day, garlic is a good energy tonic because its aromatic properties help increase circulation.

1 large eggplant, unpeeled, cut
   into 8 slices
2 teaspoons olive oil
½ teaspoon good-quality paprika

½ cup vegetable stock
Pinch of sea salt
16 cloves garlic, unpeeled
8 sprigs flat-leaf Italian parsley

*If the weather is damp:
Add hot pepper sauce to
taste to the stock mixture
before brushing it over the
eggplant slices.*

*If the weather is dry: Serve
with a juicy, ripe tomato
salad.*

Preheat the oven to 375°F. Lightly oil a glass baking dish.

Arrange the eggplant slices in the baking dish in a single layer. In a small bowl,
combine the olive oil, paprika, stock, and salt, brushing the mixture evenly over
the slices. Pour the rest of the mixture into the bottom of the dish, and bake the
slices for 15 minutes.

When the time's up, add the garlic cloves to the bottom of the baking dish
and continue to bake for 15 to 20 minutes, or until the eggplant is tender and
golden-red in color. To serve, slip off and discard the skins of the garlic cloves
and smash each clove with the flat part of a knife. The garlic will be a smooth,
sweet, and nutty paste. Place 2 smashed garlic cloves on each eggplant steak
along with a parsley sprig. Serve warm or at room temperature for a lunch or
dinner entrée.

MAKES 4 SERVINGS; 60 CALORIES PER SERVING; 2.2 GRAMS OF FAT; 32 PERCENT OF CALORIES
FROM FAT.

eggplant moons with miso-scallion sauce

If the weather is damp: Add cayenne to taste to the miso sauce before tossing with the eggplant, and serve warm.

If the weather is dry: Serve the eggplant at room temperature atop a nest of greens.

Japanese cooks and healers hold that miso, or soybean paste, is a restorative to the entire system, helping to abate heat-induced fatigue.

2 slim purple or white Asian–type eggplant (about ½ pound)
1 tablespoon miso (any type, available at Asian markets and natural food stores)

2 tablespoons vegetable stock or water
2 scallions, minced

Cut the eggplant into ½-inch slices, then cut each in half to form half-moons. Steam the eggplant over boiling water until it's just tender, 20 to 25 minutes.

Meanwhile, in a small bowl, combine the miso, stock or water, and scallions. When the eggplant is ready, tip it into a medium serving bowl, pour on the miso sauce, and toss well to combine. Serve warm or at room temperature.

MAKES 4 SIDE SERVINGS OR 2 ENTRÉE SERVINGS; 67 CALORIES PER ENTRÉE SERVING; NO ADDED FAT.

cucumber
coolest of them all

Parched and cranky one noon in Cairo, I was served a simple and delightfully rejuvenating salad of diced cucumbers seasoned with radish, onion, parsley, and lemon. One bite told me there was hope for my mood, and after enjoying the entire salad I was completely refreshed.

Mine is not the first cucumber revival story. In Chinese mythology, Li Tieh-kuai, one of the eight Chinese Immortals, tied a cucumber charm to his magic staff and from it clouds of vapor rose to free his spirit. In Hebrew myth, cucumbers and gourds are associated with renewal. Ancient legends of Burma tell of Yatawn and Yatai, tadpolelike beings who, after nibbling on a cucumber, had a passionate romance, thereupon spawning the entire Indo-Chinese race.

On a more practical note, the internal temperature of a cucumber can be as much as 20 degrees cooler than outside air—good news on a hot day. Press slices of mashed pulp onto hot, itchy rashes or burns to cool and soothe the skin. Or snack on a cuke to cool yourself internally. A seven-inch specimen contains 20 calories and no fat, plus small amounts of vitamin C, folate, and potassium. And because of their high water content, cucumbers are a natural diuretic, helping to expel excess sodium from the body—an apt antidote to salty summer junk foods.

quick cooking tips for cucumbers

For extra-fancy slices, score the peel of a cucumber lengthwise with the tines of a fork before slicing. Serve sliced cucumber in relish trays, with hummus, or spread with smoked salmon or whitefish pâté.

cucumber salad with sesame and chives

If the weather is damp: Increase the garlic to 2 cloves.

If the weather is dry: This salad is perfect.

This refreshing dish can help avert summer fatigue, thanks to the stimulating and aromatic properties of garlic and gingerroot.

4 cucumbers, seeded and thinly sliced
2 tablespoons lemon juice
1 clove garlic, mashed through a press

1 teaspoon chopped fresh chives
1 tablespoon soy sauce
½ teaspoon finely minced fresh gingerroot
½ teaspoon toasted (dark) sesame oil

In a medium bowl, combine the cucumbers, lemon juice, garlic, chives, soy sauce, and gingerroot. Let the salad marinate, covered and refrigerated, for 2 hours. Stir in the sesame oil just before serving. Great slightly chilled or at room temperature, as a lunch or dinner side dish.

MAKES 4 SERVINGS; 36 CALORIES PER SERVING; .5 GRAM OF FAT; 21 PERCENT OF CALORIES FROM FAT.

chopped cool cucumber salad

Cucumbers and tomatoes become a revitalizing summer tonic with the addition of digestion-soothing oregano. Take this dish to a summer picnic.

6 or 7 cucumbers, chopped into ½-inch pieces

1 or 2 tomatoes, chopped (juice too)

1 tablespoon balsamic vinegar

1 tablespoon minced fresh oregano

Pinch of sea salt

Freshly ground black pepper to taste

If the weather is damp: Toss in a clove of minced garlic when combining the salad.

If the weather is dry: Substitute minced fresh mint for the oregano.

In a medium bowl, combine all of the ingredients. Serve at room temperature or very slightly chilled as a lunch or dinner salad.

MAKES 4 SERVINGS; 45 CALORIES PER SERVING; NO ADDED FAT.

cucumber raita

If the weather is damp: Substitute a spicy jalapeño pepper for the mild green chile, and add freshly ground black pepper when adding the salt.

If the weather is dry: This is a perfect dish.

The cucumbers, yogurt, and cilantro make this a classic cool accompaniment to such spicy foods as Indian curries.

6 or 7 cucumbers, peeled
½ teaspoon cuminseed
½ teaspoon coriander seed
2 cups plain nonfat yogurt
3 scallions, minced
1 tomato, seeded, juiced, and chopped

1 mild green chile, seeded and minced
1 tablespoon minced fresh cilantro
Pinch of sea salt

Using a medium grater, shred the cucumbers and place in a sieve to drain for about 30 minutes.

Meanwhile, toss the cuminseed and coriander seed into a dry sauté pan on medium-high, stirring frequently until the seeds are fragrant and toasted, 2 to 3 minutes. Crush the seeds in a mortar or spice grinder.

Use your hand to press the excess liquid out of the cucumber shreds, then toss them into a medium bowl along with the yogurt, crushed seeds, scallions, tomato, chile, cilantro, and salt. Serve at room temperature or slightly chilled atop or beside spicy entrées. If the raita is stored in the fridge, stir the mixture before serving.

MAKES 6 SERVINGS; 72 CALORIES PER SERVING; NO ADDED FAT.

ocean salad

This refreshing dish is a popular summer cooler in the Hawaiian Islands and in Japan. For those who are new to eating nutritious seaweed, this is a mild and tasty introduction.

½ cup dried arame seaweed (available at Asian markets and natural food stores)

3 cucumbers, peeled, seeded, and thinly sliced

3 scallions, minced

½ teaspoon hot pepper sauce, or to taste

1 teaspoon toasted (dark) sesame oil

1 teaspoon sesame seeds

If the weather is damp: Increase the hot pepper sauce.

If the weather is dry: The salad is perfect.

In a bowl, soak the arame in hot water until tender, about 20 minutes. Drain and pat dry. Toss the arame into a medium bowl along with the cucumbers, scallions, hot pepper sauce, and sesame oil.

Tip the sesame seeds into a dry sauté pan and heat on medium-high, stirring constantly, until they're toasted, about 2 minutes. Add to the salad and toss well. Serve as a starter or side dish for lunch or dinner.

MAKES 4 SERVINGS; 51 CALORIES PER SERVING; 1 GRAM OF FAT; 26 PERCENT OF CALORIES FROM FAT.

kim chee

If the weather is damp: Add a pinch of cayenne before serving.

If the weather is dry: Mix a serving of kim chee with a cup of cooked linguine or flat rice noodles.

This spicy, lightly pickled vegetable dish is a prized body balancer for hot seasons in Korea. It is customarily served atop a bowl of steaming breakfast rice, but it can also be enjoyed as a side dish for lunch or dinner.

1 medium head (about 1½ pounds) bok choy cabbage, thinly sliced

6 or 7 cucumbers, seeded and thinly sliced

1 tablespoon sea salt

2 tablespoons soy sauce

1 tablespoon nam pla, or Asian fish sauce (available at Asian markets)

12 ounces daikon radish, thinly sliced

1 pear, grated

7 scallions, minced

4 large cloves garlic, minced

2 tablespoons grated fresh gingerroot

1 carrot, grated

1 tablespoon hot pepper sauce, or to taste

In a 4-quart bowl, combine the bok choy, cucumbers, salt, soy sauce, and nam pla. Cover with waxed paper and press the mixture for 1 hour by weighting it with a heavy object such as an iron or a cast-iron skillet. Drain away the liquids, then add the remaining ingredients. Cover the kim chee and let it marinate, refrigerated, for 24 hours before serving.

The kim chee will keep, covered and refrigerated, for about 2 weeks. Try it as a condiment instead of the usual dill pickle.

MAKES ABOUT 3 QUARTS, OR TWENTY-FOUR ½-CUP SERVINGS; 25 CALORIES PER SERVING; NO ADDED FAT.

cucumber sun pickles

Summer sun "cooks" these tasty spears, perfuming them with stomach-soothing dillweed. In addition, the gentle taste is appealing to children.

4 to 6 cucumbers, sliced into spears
About 2 cups cider vinegar
Pinch of sea salt, or to taste

2 sprigs fresh dillweed
2 cloves garlic, chopped

Pack the spears vertically into a glass jar and cover with the vinegar. Add the salt, dillweed, and garlic, and cover the jar. Let the jar sit in sunlight, on a windowsill or outside, for 2 days. Store refrigerated.

MAKES ABOUT 8 SERVINGS; 7.5 CALORIES PER SERVING; NO ADDED FAT.

If the weather is damp: Serve the pickles as an accompaniment to a spicy dish.

If the weather is dry: Serve the pickles on a relish tray with juicy, ripe tomatoes.

cucumber freezer pickles

Cucumbers and shallots remain crisp and succulent with this innovative and cool pickling method. Make them now, and enjoy them later.

4 or 5 cucumbers, thinly sliced
1 shallot, thinly sliced
About 1 cup white vinegar
¼ cup honey

2 cloves garlic, sliced
Pinch of sea salt
8 sprigs fresh dillweed

In a 1-quart freezer container, layer the cukes and shallot.

In a medium bowl, whisk together the vinegar, honey, garlic, and salt. Arrange the dillweed atop the cucumbers and pour on the vinegar mixture, leaving about ½ inch of head space. Add more vinegar if necessary. Cover the container and freeze for up to 3 months. Defrost overnight in the refrigerator.

MAKES 1 QUART, OR EIGHT ½-CUP SERVINGS; 50 CALORIES PER SERVING; NO ADDED FAT.

If the weather is damp: Add 1 teaspoon each mustard seed and peppercorns to the vinegar mixture.

If the weather is dry: Add 2 teaspoons allspice berries to the vinegar mixture.

sesame cucumbers with sushi rice

If the weather is damp: Substitute hot chili oil for the sesame oil and serve warm or at room temperature.

If the weather is dry: Serve slightly chilled on a bed of crisp mixed greens.

This revitalizing dish is a good introduction to the Japanese art of sushi, or vinegared rice.

1 cup short-grain Japanese-style rice	1 cucumber, julienned
1¼ cups water	2 tablespoons toasted sesame seeds
1 tablespoon rice vinegar	2 scallions, finely minced
1 tablespoon mirin (sweet rice vinegar) or sherry	1 teaspoon toasted (dark) sesame oil

Rinse the rice, then combine it in a medium saucepan with the water and let it sit for 30 minutes. Then bring the water to a boil, reduce the heat immediately, and simmer the rice, stirring frequently, until all of the water has been absorbed, 10 to 12 minutes.

Remove the rice from the heat and stir in the remaining ingredients. Serve at room temperature or very slightly chilled as a lunch or dinner entrée.

MAKES 4 SERVINGS; 220 CALORIES PER SERVING; 3 GRAMS OF FAT; 14 PERCENT OF CALORIES FROM FAT.

minted cucumber ice

If the weather is damp: Garnish with cinnamon-scented toasted oat granola.

If the weather is dry: The recipe is perfect.

Revitalizing mint unites with bracing cucumber and cantaloupe to make a tinglingly cool summer dessert.

1 cup brewed, cooled mint tea	½ medium cantaloupe, cubed
⅓ cup honey	2 tablespoons lemon juice
4 or 5 cucumbers, peeled, halved, and seeded	

In a food processor or blender, combine all of the ingredients and process until smooth. Add to an ice cream maker and proceed according to the manufacturer's instructions. Serve immediately.

MAKES ABOUT 3 CUPS, OR SIX ½-CUP SERVINGS; 65 CALORIES PER SERVING; NO ADDED FAT.

zucchini
the sociable squash

One election year, while waiting in line to mail a package, I saw this written on light blue construction paper, taped to a wall:

"If I were Presdent I would wish for a better world. And no gun's or wars. NO litter. And every boty would be friend's. And noboty would lie. No boty would eat brussel sprouts or zewkeine. Brad F. age 7."

I could imagine Brad F. at the dinner table complaining about the boring "zewkeine." But zucchini's bland taste is exactly what makes it so great to cook with. Zucchini is hospitable to surrounding flavors—few other vegetables can so easily take in the tastes and aromas around them. Be it garlic, gingerroot, tarragon, thyme, Italian cuisine, Thai, Mexican, or Japanese, zucchini works. That means no taste clashes, and very easy cooking.

Zucchini's ability to readily harmonize with other flavors made it popular in its native Italy, where the word *zucchini* means "little squash." In England it is called "marrow," and the French say *courgette* for "little gourd." Zucchini made its print debut in the United States in the February 1929 issue of *Sunset* magazine, where it was spelled "succini," and the recipe called for it to be baked in a casserole with tomato sauce, onion, garlic, and cheeses. It was an instant hit.

Gardeners, too, love zucchini, because its rapid growth makes them look like wonder gardeners. It's not a case of cultivation expertise: The veggies swell so rapidly due to an extremely high water content, making them a hydrating and refreshing summer vegetable. Half a cup of cooked zucchini contains 18 calories and virtually no fat—yet another hot-weather bonus.

flower power

Zucchini blossoms can be stuffed with rice mixtures or with chopped vegetable salads, then served as is or lightly sautéed. If you're gleaning the blossoms from your garden, be sure to pick only the males (they're the ones with the long, narrow stems, as opposed to the females, which have rounder stems). This way the plant will continue to produce.

quick cooking tips for zucchini

Coarsely grate zucchini into a coleslaw recipe, substituting it for half of the cabbage; slice it into batons and use on a relish tray, or to scoop garlicky dips.

refrigerator zucchini pickles

Celery seed, turmeric, and mustard all contain magnesium, a mineral that when introduced into the diet can help alleviate summer fatigue and headaches.

3 to 4 medium zucchini, thinly
   sliced (about 1 pound)
1 onion, thinly sliced
2 cloves garlic, sliced
1 cup cider vinegar
2 tablespoons honey

2 teaspoons celery seed
1 teaspoon ground turmeric
½ teaspoon dry mustard
1 teaspoon mustard seed
Pinch of sea salt

In a glass jar, arrange the zucchini, onion, and garlic.

In a small saucepan, combine the remaining ingredients and heat gently, don't boil. Pour the mixture over the vegetables and let it sit for 1 hour. Cover and place in the refrigerator, where the pickles will last for a month.

MAKES ABOUT 2 CUPS, OR EIGHT ¼-CUP SERVINGS; 35 CALORIES PER SERVING; NO ADDED FAT.

If the weather is damp: Serve the pickles on a relish tray, along with spicy salsa and baked tortilla chips.

If the weather is dry: Pack the pickles into a sandwich with fresh sliced tomatoes.

zucchini with tomato and garlic

If the weather is damp: Serve warm atop crusty bread slices.

If the weather is dry: Toss with just-cooked linguine.

Oregano serves to perfume this dish, as well as to soothe a stressed summer mood. It's a great fast summer dish that won't heat up the kitchen.

1 shallot, minced
2 cloves garlic, minced
¼ cup vegetable stock or water
3 average zucchini, thinly sliced
2 large tomatoes, peeled, seeded, and chopped

Pinch of sea salt
1 tablespoon minced fresh oregano, or 1½ teaspoons dried

In a large sauté pan, combine the shallot, garlic, and stock. Heat on high for about a minute, then add the zucchini, tomatoes, and salt (if you're using dry oregano, add it now), sautéing until the zucchini is just tender and the tomatoes are saucy, 3 to 4 minutes (if you're using fresh oregano, stir it in now). Serve warm, at room temperature, or very slightly chilled as a side dish to grilled fish.

MAKES 4 SERVINGS; 45 CALORIES PER SERVING; NO ADDED FAT.

zucchini "pasta" with fresh basil

According to ancient Ayurvedic texts, basil can cool and soothe an irritable summer mood. The herb also contains aromatic compounds that can help alleviate irritable digestion.

1 cup vegetable stock
2 cloves garlic, minced
1 carrot, julienned
4 large zucchini, sliced into ⅛-inch linguinelike strips (that's the "pasta"!)

¼ cup grated Parmesan cheese or soy Parmesan
¼ cup grated low-fat mozzarella or soy mozzarella
¼ cup regular or soy milk
¼ cup minced fresh basil

If the weather is damp: Add a pinch of cayenne when stirring in the basil.

If the weather is dry: Add a chopped fresh tomato when stirring in the basil.

In a large sauté pan, combine the stock and garlic and heat on high until slightly reduced, 1 to 2 minutes. Reduce the heat to medium and add the carrot. Cover and cook for about 3 minutes. Then add the zucchini, cover, and continue to cook until the vegetables are tender, 1 to 2 minutes. Drain the liquid and toss in the Parmesan, mozzarella, milk, and basil. Serve immediately as a lunch or dinner entrée.

MAKES 4 SERVINGS; 100 CALORIES PER SERVING; 3 GRAMS OF FAT; 27 PERCENT OF CALORIES FROM FAT.

zucchini milk

If the weather is damp: Use zucchini milk as the base for a spicy summer vegetable soup.

If the weather is dry: Use zucchini milk as the base for chilled tomato soup.

For those who have summer colds and allergies, especially when residing or working in polluted areas, Chinese and Ayurvedic healers recommend the elimination of dairy products. This includes milk, but zucchini provides an interesting alternative.

4 very fresh medium zucchini

Peel the zucchini and cut into chunks. Toss the chunks into a food processor or blender and process until liquefied. This is zucchini milk.

Use it to replace dairy milk in summer ice cream recipes, puddings, creamy pie and tart fillings, casseroles, soups, stews, muffins, waffles, quick breads, and even morning oatmeal. Zucchini milk will keep, frozen, for up to 6 months.

MAKES ABOUT 2 CUPS; 20 CALORIES PER ½ CUP; NO ADDED FAT.

thyme-braised summer vegetables

This light stew has a top note of thyme, an herb that French healers say fights hot weather fatigue. The dish keeps well, so you may wish to pack it to take to work for lunch.

2 zucchini, chopped

2 yellow summer squash, chopped

1 medium onion, chopped

1 large eggplant, chopped

2 red or yellow bell peppers, cored, seeded, and chopped

1 pound tomatoes, cored and chopped

3 cloves garlic, minced

1 bay leaf

1 tablespoon minced fresh thyme, or 1½ teaspoons dried

Pinch of sea salt

Freshly ground black pepper to taste

If the weather is damp: Add a minced jalapeño along with the rest of the ingredients and serve the stew warm, garnished with crisp croutons.

If the weather is dry: Serve the stew slightly chilled, sprinkled with minced fresh mint.

In a large stockpot, combine all of the ingredients and bring to a boil. Reduce the heat to medium-low, cover loosely, and simmer until the vegetables are fragrant and tender, about 35 minutes. Stir occasionally. Serve warm or slightly chilled as a starter with crusty whole wheat bread, or as a side dish.

MAKES 4 SERVINGS; 62 CALORIES PER SERVING; NO ADDED FAT.

rosemary-scented zucchini

If the weather is damp: Add hot pepper sauce to taste to the filling before scooping it into the shells.

If the weather is dry: Serve with a salad of fresh ripe tomatoes that have been tossed with balsamic vinegar.

Rosemary's aromatic properties can refresh and rejuvenate the weary. In addition, if you use brown rice, the B vitamins it offers will help soothe the nervous system.

2 medium zucchini, each about 7 inches long

2 shallots, minced

½ cup cooked rice

1 medium tomato, chopped

¼ cup vegetable stock or water

2 teaspoons minced fresh rosemary

1 clove garlic, minced

Pinch of sea salt

Freshly ground black pepper to taste

Preheat the oven to 350°F.

Slice the zucchini lengthwise. Using a grapefruit spoon, scoop out the flesh and keep it handy, leaving a ¼-inch-thick shell.

Mince the zucchini flesh and tip it into a large sauté pan along with the remaining ingredients. Heat on medium-high until the mixture is fragrant and saucy and the vegetables are just tender, about 6 minutes.

Scoop the filling into the zucchini shells and arrange them in a lightly oiled baking pan. Cover and bake until fragrant and warmed through for about 25 minutes, then chill in the fridge. Serve very slightly chilled as a lunch or dinner entrée.

MAKES 4 SERVINGS; 70 CALORIES PER SERVING; NO ADDED FAT.

fruits
cool feast in the heat

In La Cieba, Honduras, I learned a tale of trees, in which friendly spirits flutter out of the branches at night to keep watch and ensure that all is well. One of their jobs, should you believe the story, is to protect the fruit crops. People in Honduras rely on the high water content in fresh fruit to stay cool and hydrated in the heat. Eating sliced succulent mangoes, mouthwatering melons, berries, plums, peaches, cherries, and other luscious offerings can keep you refreshed as well. In addition, most fruits provide a good amount of the skin-enhancing nutrients vitamin C and beta carotene—a protective repast when basking in summer sun.

sweet and sour

Summer stone fruits, such as peaches, plums, nectarines, and cherries, make beautiful and tasty homemade vinegars: Pile your choice of peach peels, plum slices, pitted halved cherries, or nectarine slices in a small saucepan. Pour on cider vinegar to cover and bring up the heat to medium. Simmer, don't boil, for about five minutes. Let the vinegar cool with the fruit in it, then discard the fruit and bottle the vinegar. Use summer fruit vinegar in salad dressings, marinades, and sauces. Or, for a tasty and revitalizing beverage, mix one teaspoon of the fruit vinegar in one cup of seltzer water and serve in a chilled glass garnished with fresh mint.

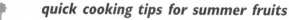

quick cooking tips for summer fruits

For quick energy and hydration in summer heat, add sliced peaches or grapes to green salads, toss plum wedges with chicken salad, slice nectarines over pancakes or waffles before serving, dot a lemon or vanilla mousse with fresh berries and cherries.

cantaloupe in lime-ginger syrup

If the weather is damp: Add a pinch of ground cinnamon to the syrup before simmering.

If the weather is dry: This dessert is perfect.

This bracing dessert is an instant digestive tonic, thanks to the aromatic properties of the fresh gingerroot.

Juice of 1 lime, plus lime zest for
   garnish
²/₃ cup orange juice
5 slices fresh gingerroot

¼ cup honey
1 cantaloupe, peeled, seeded, and
   cut into chunks

In a small saucepan, combine the lime juice, orange juice, gingerroot, and honey and bring to a boil. Reduce the heat to medium and simmer, uncovered, until the syrup thickens, 12 to 15 minutes.

In a large bowl, combine the hot syrup and cantaloupe chunks, cover, and refrigerate until cold, at least an hour. Serve in chilled martini glasses garnished with the lime zest.

MAKES 4 SERVINGS; 90 CALORIES PER SERVING; NO ADDED FAT.

raspberries in balsamic honey

Succulent raspberries are made even more bracing with the addition of a honey-sweetened balsamic vinegar marinade.

2 pints raspberries

2 tablespoons light honey, such as wildflower or orange

1 tablespoon balsamic vinegar

Mint leaves for garnish

Place the berries in a large glass bowl. In a small bowl, whisk together the honey and vinegar and pour it over the berries. Toss well but gently to combine. Cover and refrigerate for about an hour, then serve in chilled dessert bowls garnished with the mint.

MAKES 4 SERVINGS; 97 CALORIES PER SERVING; NO ADDED FAT.

If the weather is damp: Serve with crisp cookies.

If the weather is dry: This dessert is perfect.

peaches in honey wine

For extra summer refreshment, be sure to use freestone peaches in this recipe. The flesh is juicier than clingstone types, and of course, the pits are easier to remove.

5 peaches, pitted and sliced

2/3 cup red wine (or apple juice if you're not drinking)

3 tablespoons honey (omit if using apple juice)

One 2-inch piece of lemon zest

Toss the peaches into a large glass bowl. In a medium bowl, whisk together the wine and honey and pour it over the peaches. Toss well but gently to combine, adding the lemon zest as you go. Chill for at least 20 minutes before serving for a dessert or refreshing snack.

MAKES 4 SERVINGS; 189 CALORIES PER SERVING; NO ADDED FAT.

If the weather is damp: Add a pinch of ground cinnamon to the wine before tossing with the peaches.

If the weather is dry: This dessert is perfect.

peach salad with walnut vinaigrette

If the weather is damp: Be generous with the black pepper.

If the weather is dry: The salad is perfect.

Peaches and watercress combine to quench a parched palate. What's more, peaches are a good source of beta carotene, a boost for summer skin health.

1 Belgian endive, separated into petals

4 ripe peaches, peeled, pitted, and sliced

2 scallions, minced

2 tablespoons chopped toasted walnuts

Watercress for garnish

1 tablespoon walnut oil

2 tablespoons lemon juice

1 tablespoon balsamic vinegar

Pinch of sea salt

Freshly ground black pepper to taste

On a chilled serving plate, arrange the endive petals in a spoke pattern. Arrange the peach slices atop the endive. Sprinkle with the scallions and walnuts and garnish with the cress.

In a small bowl, whisk together the walnut oil, lemon juice, vinegar, salt, and pepper and sprinkle over the salad. Serve as a side dish or as a starter for lunch or dinner.

MAKES 4 SERVINGS; 120 CALORIES PER SERVING; 5.5 GRAMS OF FAT; 41 PERCENT OF CALORIES FROM FAT.

cinnamon-peach cobbler

Depending on availability, you may wish to substitute other hydrating fruits such as plums, nectarines, cherries, or berries for the peaches in this cobbler.

If the weather is damp: Serve the cobbler warm.

If the weather is dry: Serve the cobbler slightly chilled.

2 egg whites, or ¼ cup commercial
   egg substitute
¼ cup pure maple syrup
1 tablespoon canola oil
⅓ cup buttermilk or low-fat
   soy milk

½ cup whole wheat pastry flour
2 teaspoons baking powder
3 cups peeled, pitted, and sliced
   peaches (from about 2 pounds)
1 teaspoon ground cinnamon
1 teaspoon cornstarch

Preheat the oven to 375°F. Lightly oil an 8-inch-square baking pan.

In a medium bowl, combine the egg whites or egg substitute, maple syrup, oil, and milk and whisk until well combined. In another medium bowl, combine the flour and baking powder. Pour the egg white mixture into the flour mixture and combine well but don't overmix. About 12 strokes should do it.

In another bowl, combine the peaches, cinnamon, and cornstarch. Tip them into the prepared baking pan. Spread the batter evenly over the peach mixture and bake until fragrant, crisp, and golden, 18 to 20 minutes. Serve warm or slightly chilled for breakfast, brunch, or dessert.

MAKES 6 SERVINGS; 190 CALORIES PER SERVING; 2.3 GRAMS OF FAT; 10 PERCENT OF CALORIES FROM FAT.

plum preserves

If the weather is damp:
Add a 2-inch cinnamon
stick to the boiling
preserves and discard
before jarring.

Plums offer immune-boosting vitamin C, as well as the cancer-fighting substance ellagic acid. They are also a good source of digestion-toning insoluble fiber—a tasty alternative to prunes.

If the weather is dry:
Spread the preserves on a
moist banana muffin for
breakfast.

1 pound ripe plums, pitted and chopped (including juice)
½ lemon, seeded and minced (including peel)

½ cup honey

In a large saucepan, combine all of the ingredients and bring to a boil. Continue to boil and stir until the mixture is thick and jamlike, a bit darker, and slightly translucent, 15 to 20 minutes. Let the preserves cool slightly before jarring and refrigerating for up to a month. Spread on toast or pancakes.

MAKES 1 CUP OR EIGHT 2-TABLESPOON SERVINGS; 88 CALORIES PER SERVING; NO ADDED FAT.

sweet and sour sauce

If the weather is damp:
Add ground ginger to taste
before simmering, and
serve warm with grilled
fish or grilled vegetables.

In Chinese healing theory, eating sweet tastes can help you feel relaxed, while sour tastes can help you focus. This recipe combines both attributes.

If the weather is dry: Use
as a sauce with stir-fried
vegetables.

¾ cup plum preserves (above) or buy a naturally sweetened brand
¾ cup naturally sweetened apricot preserves

½ cup cider vinegar
1 teaspoon balsamic vinegar
1 allspice berry, ground
Pinch of sea salt

In a medium saucepan, combine all of the ingredients and bring to a boil. Immediately lower the heat to a simmer and continue cooking and stirring until the mixture thickens, about 10 minutes. Serve as a condiment with spring rolls, grilled tofu, or spicy grilled fish.

MAKES 1 CUP, OR FOUR ¼-CUP SERVINGS; 271 CALORIES PER SERVING; NO ADDED FAT.

frozen cherry yogurt

As a good source of potassium, cherries can help prevent sodium-induced high blood pressure from those summer junk foods.

2 cups pitted, chopped cherries with their juice
2 cups plain nonfat yogurt

1/3 cup honey
1/2 teaspoon pure vanilla extract

In a food processor or blender, combine all of the ingredients and process until smooth. Pour the mixture into an ice cream maker and proceed according to the manufacturer's instructions. Serve immediately.

MAKES 4 CUPS, OR 4 LARGE SERVINGS; 107 CALORIES PER SERVING; NO ADDED FAT.

If the weather is damp: Add 1/2 teaspoon ground cinnamon to the mixture before processing.

If the weather is dry: Garnish with fresh pitted cherries.

blueberry-ginger sorbet

This icy dessert is a summer digestive tonic for two reasons: The blueberries are a good source of dietary fiber, and the gingerroot contains compounds that soothe heat-induced indigestion.

1 pint fresh blueberries
1/4 cup honey
2 tablespoons lemon juice

One 6-ounce bottle of naturally sweetened ginger ale

In a food processor or blender, combine the blueberries, honey, and lemon juice and process until pureed. Stir in the ginger ale and pour the mixture into an ice cream maker. Proceed according to the manufacturer's instructions. Serve immediately.

MAKES 4 SERVINGS; 130 CALORIES PER SERVING; NO ADDED FAT.

If the weather is damp: Add 1/2 teaspoon grated fresh gingerroot to the mixture before processing.

If the weather is dry: Garnish with whole fresh berries.

fresh raspberry slush

If the weather is damp:
Add a dash of lemon zest
before blending.

If the weather is dry: This
recipe is perfect.

This invigorating dessert or snack is a great summer health potion, containing such immune-boosting nutrients as vitamin C and folate, as well as the nerve-toning B vitamins.

About a half pint red raspberries   **1 teaspoon lemon juice**
½ cup white grape juice   **1½ cups crushed ice**

In a blender, combine all of the ingredients and whiz until very well combined and slushy. Serve immediately.

MAKES 2 SERVINGS; 102 CALORIES PER SERVING; NO ADDED FAT.

lemon-berry ice cream

If the weather is damp:
Garnish with minced
candied ginger.

If the weather is dry: This
recipe is perfect.

Japanese healers hold that lemon is a liver tonic and that imbibing it regularly can soothe such heat-induced conditions as irritability and even jealousy.

1½ pints fresh berries of   **½ teaspoon finely grated lemon zest**
    your choice   **1 cup skim, low-fat soy, whole milk,**
½ cup honey   **or cream**
¼ cup lemon juice

Tip the berries, honey, lemon juice, and lemon zest into a food processor or blender and process until smooth. If you're using raspberries and wish to eliminate the seeds, press the mixture through a fine sieve.

Stir in the milk and add to an ice cream maker, proceeding according to the manufacturer's instructions. Serve immediately.

MAKES 4 SERVINGS; 100 CALORIES PER SERVING; NO ADDED FAT.

mint-marinated pineapple

Ayurvedic healers say that pineapple is a summer restorative for all types of people, calming and cooling heat-provoked gastritis.

1 fresh pineapple, cut into 1-inch chunks

3 tablespoons crème de menthe, or ¼ cup lime juice

Fresh mint leaves for garnish

If the weather is damp: Serve with gingersnap cookies.

If the weather is dry: This recipe is perfect.

In a glass bowl, combine the pineapple and crème de menthe or lime juice, cover, and refrigerate for an hour. Serve chilled in chilled wineglasses, garnished with the mint leaves, for dessert.

MAKES 4 SERVINGS; 115 CALORIES PER SERVING; NO ADDED FAT.

tofu
refreshing inside and out

One morning while studying Japanese cooking, I entered my instructor's kitchen and found her applying a mashed tofu poultice to a burn on her hand. Tofu, she explained, is so cooling that it actually draws heat from external burns. It does the same internally, she continued, cooling and soothing "hot" stomach and digestive distresses.

For nutrition particulars, four ounces of regular tofu contain about 120 calories, 54 percent of which come from fat. Low-fat tofu contains about 80 calories for the same amount, about 30 percent of which come from fat.

tofu types

When shopping for tofu, most of what you will find is the traditional firm Chinese type, adaptable to all recipes. Some natural food stores and supermarkets offer a "soft" type of tofu that's particularly easy to blend into dips and spreads; and an "extra firm" type that holds its shape well when stir-fried. Be sure to buy tofu that smells fresh and slightly nutty. If it smells sour, it's old and shouldn't be eaten. If tofu is packaged and you can't smell it, check the expiration date on the label.

❋ **quick cooking tips for tofu**

The creamy white blocks can be sliced, marinated in soy sauce and sesame seeds, and grilled; or blanched (slice and simmer in water for two minutes) and pureed to fill in for sour cream in dip recipes. For the best digestion, always be sure to cook tofu before eating it.

kung fu tofu
(tofu spread with a kick)

Though this recipe is based on cooling tofu, the onion, garlic, chives, cayenne, and gingerroot help balance the "cold" nature of the dish, aiding in increasing circulation in the body.

1 pound low-fat tofu, crumbled	Pinch of cayenne, or to taste
2 tablespoons grated onion	1 teaspoon grated fresh gingerroot
1 clove garlic, minced	1 teaspoon toasted (dark) sesame oil
1 tablespoon minced fresh chives	2 teaspoons tahini (sesame butter)
1 large tomato, chopped	Pinch of sea salt
1 to 2 teaspoons hot pepper sauce	1 teaspoon soy sauce

If the weather is damp: Spread the tofu on crusty bread as an appetizer, snack, or sandwich. Or use to garnish a spicy chili dish.

If the weather is dry: Toss 1/4 cup of the tofu spread with 1 cup just-cooked pasta and garnish with minced fresh tomato.

Steam the tofu and onion over boiling water for about 4 minutes. Then toss into a food processor or blender with the rest of the ingredients and process until smooth. Serve as a sandwich spread, or as a dip for sliced cucumbers and carrot sticks.

MAKES 2½ CUPS, OR TEN ¼-CUP SERVINGS; 58 CALORIES PER SERVING; 2 GRAMS OF FAT; 30 PERCENT OF CALORIES FROM FAT.

tofu-basil spread

If the weather is damp:
Add a pinch of cayenne, or
to taste, to the mixture
before processing.

———

If the weather is dry:
Spread on cucumber or
zucchini rounds and serve
as an appetizer.

The uplifting flavor of basil—combining mint, cloves, and thyme—is a soothing summer refresher. The pleasant and familiar taste of the herb makes this recipe a good introduction for tofu novices.

½ pound low-fat tofu, crumbled

2 to 3 cloves garlic, minced

2 tomatoes, chopped

2 cups fresh basil leaves

1 tablespoon olive oil

2 tablespoons grated Parmesan
cheese or soy Parmesan

1 teaspoon prepared mustard

Steam the tofu and garlic over boiling water for 4 minutes. Then combine in a food processor or blender with the remaining ingredients and process until smooth. Serve at room temperature or slightly chilled as a spread for crusty bread, or atop fresh tomato slices.

MAKES ABOUT 2 CUPS, OR EIGHT ¼-CUP SERVINGS; 61 CALORIES PER SERVING; 3 GRAMS OF FAT; 43 PERCENT OF CALORIES FROM FAT.

rose and almond spread

If the weather is damp:
Spead on cinnamon toast
and serve for breakfast.

———

If the weather is dry:
Spread on a banana muffin
and serve for breakfast.

Ayurvedic healers say that rose and almond are calming and fortifying to a heat-stressed mind and body.

½ pound low-fat tofu, crumbled

2 tablespoons almond butter

1 teaspoon rosewater

1 teaspoon lemon juice

Steam the tofu over boiling water for 4 minutes. Then combine the tofu in a food processor or blender with the almond butter, rosewater, and lemon juice and process until smooth. Serve at room temperature or very slightly chilled, spread on a muffin or toast.

MAKES 1½ CUPS, OR SIX ¼-CUP SERVINGS; 75 CALORIES PER SERVING; 3.8 GRAMS OF FAT; 42 PERCENT OF CALORIES FROM FAT.

smiling tofu

This traditional Chinese summer recipe is cooling to the body and spirit—and if you're wondering why the recipe is so named, it's because the marinated, stuffed tofu makes little grins when filled.

If the weather is damp: Serve the tofu warm, sprinkled with freshly ground black pepper.

If the weather is dry: Serve the tofu slightly chilled and substitute minced fresh cilantro for the chives.

For the Marinade:
- 1 tablespoon soy sauce
- 1 tablespoon mirin (sweet rice vinegar) or sherry
- 1 teaspoon toasted (dark) sesame oil
- 2 slices gingerroot, minced
- 1 clove garlic, minced
- ⅓ cup vegetable stock

For the Tofu:
- One 1-pound block firm, low-fat tofu
- ⅓ cup corn kernels, minced
- 3 scallions, minced
- ½ teaspoon minced fresh gingerroot
- 1 clove garlic, minced
- ½ teaspoon toasted (dark) sesame oil
- ¼ cup water chestnuts, minced
- 1½ teaspoons cornstarch
- ⅔ cup vegetable stock
- 2 tablespoons minced fresh chives

In a shallow dish, combine all of the marinade ingredients.

Slice an X through the tofu block, forming 4 equal triangles. Cut each triangle horizontally, making 8 triangles. To make pockets for the filling, slice each triangle horizontally (beginning at a point), stopping about ½ inch before you get to the end. Soak the triangles in the marinade for 20 minutes, 10 minutes on each side.

In a food processor or blender, combine the corn, scallions, gingerroot, garlic, sesame oil, water chestnuts, cornstarch, and a tablespoon of the marinade and process until combined.

Divide the filling into 8 equal portions and gently stuff the triangles, smoothing off the filled edges with your finger. See them smile?

Preheat a large, well-seasoned cast-iron pan (or a lightly oiled nonstick sauté pan) on medium-high and add the triangles on their filled edges. Sizzle for 1 minute on each filled edge and 1 minute on each flat side. Add the stock and simmer for 6 minutes, flipping the triangles midway. (If your pan's not large enough, cook 4 triangles at a time.) Remove the triangles to a serving tray. Then add the marinade to the pan, increase the heat to high, and reduce the liquid by half. Pour over the triangles and sprinkle with the chives. Serve as a lunch or dinner entrée.

MAKES 4 SERVINGS; 180 CALORIES PER SERVING; 4.75 GRAMS OF FAT; 21 PERCENT OF CALORIES FROM FAT.

IDEAS FOR COOL SUMMER MEALS

What you want to cook right now are fresh, seasonal foods that require little fuss. Quick outdoor grilling or roasting fits the season, as do chopped, raw salads. Try these tasty menus, or invent your own.

Soothing Summer Dinner: Eggplant, the entrée on which this meal is based, contains a compound called "guar gum," which can soothe a stressed stomach and indigestion. In addition, corn offers nerve-calming B vitamins; and mint acts as a refrigerant, to cool a body and mind that have become "hot tempered."

* Roasted Sweet Corn Soup with Fresh Thyme (page 166)
* Eggplant Steaks with Silky Garlic (page 183)
* Mint-Marinated Pineapple (page 209)

Easy Summer Picnic: Make the items in this menu ahead and pack them for an outing, or for your lunch break at work. Be sure to put the Minted Cucumber Ice in a freezer container so it doesn't melt. If that's impossible, pack fresh peaches and plums for dessert instead.

* Grilled Black Bean Burgers with Corn (page 167)
* Tomato Salad with Red Onion and Watercress (page 172)
* Refrigerator Zucchini Pickles (page 195)
* Minted Cucumber Ice (page 192)

Sunday Summer Brunch: This is an easy meal to prepare ahead for guests or just for yourself. To serve, chop the tomatoes and sprinkle atop the crepes.

* Fresh Corn Crepes (page 164)
* Herb-Scented Grilled Tomatoes (page 171)
* Lemon-Berry Ice Cream (page 208)

Breathe-Easy Summer Breakfast: This is the perfect way to start the day for those who have sinus trouble and allergies. Both dishes contain beta carotene, which helps stop mucus production.

* Cinnamon-Peach Cobbler (page 205)
* Cantaloupe in Lime-Ginger Syrup (page 202)

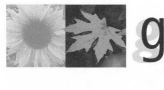

gateway
from summer
to autumn

a lthough the body's journey from one season to the next is always fascinating, no journey is more abundant with challenge than the passage from summer to autumn. As daylight subtly diminishes, so might our activity level, energy, and the stamina we need to help prevent seasonal viruses and other ailments. In fact, the summer-to-autumn transition is so critical that Chinese healers refer to it as a season of its own—the Earth season—a time to center and balance the body. "Be sympathetic to the flesh during this time," a Chinese doctor told me, and I took his words to mean that proper tending of the body and mind at this time would prepare us well for the coming seasons.

how your garden grows

Our gardens, even if they consist of just a potted plant on a windowsill, are keen metaphors of ourselves. How do we care for them? Are they lush and healthy or neglected and a bit worn? As we know this is the time of year to "be sympathetic" to ourselves, it is also prime time to care for our gardens. To prepare outdoor plants for the seasonal change, snip away and discard dying branches and leaves;

prune herbs and other perennials to sturdy, windproof shapes; mulch the bases of plants to keep the roots warm and safe. In addition, now is the time to preserve the herbal harvest, creating tea blends and other potions that will help to keep you well in the coming chillier months. If you don't grow herbs, try these techniques with those you've purchased.

Drying Herbs—Herbs dry easily in the microwave, and the flavors and colors remain livelier than if you simply hang them to dry. As an extra bonus, with the microwave method there is less risk of the herbs' molding and rotting due to unpredictable weather conditions. To try it, arrange about a cup of fresh leaves on a sheet of waxed paper right on the microwave floor. Microwave on full power, uncovered, until the leaves are dry to the touch, one to two minutes, stopping at thirty-second intervals to stir. Listen while you're stirring, and if the herbs rattle, they're dry. Let the dried herbs cool completely, then store in a covered glass jar in a cool, dry place, and they will remain flavorful for about eight months. In cooking, use one to two teaspoons in a dish to serve four, rubbing the dried herb between your hands first, to encourage fragrance. To make teas, use one teaspoon for each one-cup serving. Try mint and/or oregano as an autumn digestive tonic; basil for a blue mood; rosemary to mellow a headache; or thyme to temporarily clear upper respiratory congestion.

Herbal Vinegars—Pack about three tablespoons of fresh herbs into a one-and-a-half-cup glass jar, then pound them lightly with a spoon to bruise them and release their aromas. Heat (don't boil) one cup of cider vinegar, and pour it over the herbs. Let the vinegar cool, then cover and stash in a cool place for a couple of weeks before using in salad dressings, sauces, soups, stews, and marinades. Try basil, bay, and garlic; mint and lemon peel.

You can also add a teaspoon of herbal vinegar (omit garlic) to a half cup of distilled water and use as a skin freshener or aftershave. Store the facial tonic in the refrigerator for up to a month, splashing on after washing or shaving, before moisturizing. By adjusting the skin's pH, the tonic helps keep skin healthy and smooth during the summer-autumn transition.

Herbal Oils—Pack about three tablespoons of fresh herbs into a one-cup glass jar and pound the herbs lightly with a spoon to bruise them and release their aromas. Heat about a half cup of olive oil until it's warm, then pour over the herbs. Let the oil cool, then cover and refrigerate for a couple of weeks before using in salad dressings, marinades, or as a toss for hot vegetables. Try ginger and mint; thyme and parsley. Or, use lavender and rose to make a moisturizing facial oil for all skin types. Apply it to damp skin after washing, or while skin is moist from herbal water. Herbed oils will keep for about nine months, covered and refrigerated.

Herbal Waters—Combine a third of a cup of fresh herbs and flowers and three cups of distilled water in a glass bowl. Cover with plastic wrap and set the bowl in the sun for eight hours. Strain and use as a refreshing facial splash. Try rose, for hydrating rosewater; lavender or calendula to soothe the skin; hyssop, rosemary, or sage for oily skin. Pour the fragrant water into a spray bottle and mist as needed, especially before moisturizing. To enjoy the spray throughout the autumn and winter, freeze extra herb water in ice cube trays, transferring the cubes to plastic bags and defrosting as needed.

Herbal Skin Cleansers and Masks—For an exfoliating autumn cleanser that helps dissolve a fading summer tan, in a small jar combine equal parts of rice bran (available at natural food stores and Asian markets) and powdered milk. Add several crushed dried sprigs of lavender or calendula for normal or irritated skin; sage or rosemary for oily skin; or several dried rose petals for dry skin. To use, combine about two teaspoons of the mixture in your hand with enough water to make a paste. Rub onto your face and neck, moving your fingertips in gentle circles, for about two minutes, then rinse well and splash your face with herbal water before moisturizing with herbal oil (see above for both).

For tired or stressed skin, make a nourishing facial mask by grinding rolled oats in a blender or food processor until the oats are very fine. Combine about two tablespoons of the ground oats with one teaspoon of ground dried chamomile flowers. Mix with enough water to make a paste and apply to warm, rinsed skin. Leave on for about twenty minutes, then rinse well and follow with herbal water and herbal oil (see above for both). As a substitute for the water in the mask, for dry skin use plain yogurt or milk; for oily or irritated skin use aloe gel; for normal, dry, or dehydrated skin use honey.

Herbal Body Powders—Combine three quarters of a cup of cornstarch with a quarter cup of finely ground (use a food processor or blender) dried lavender flowers, rose petals, or rose geranium leaves: Decide what to use by what smells best to you. Store in an airtight container and sprinkle on at will. For a refreshing foot powder, use ground dried rosemary leaves.

Herbal Fatigue Fighter—Thermogenic foods, those that create "heat," help to increase circulation, thus energizing the body. Garlic is one such food, and it can be very beneficial in this sometimes gloomy time of year, especially in cases of the midafternoon blues. Try it if you feel "down" mentally or physically by wrapping a peeled clove of raw garlic in a small piece of bread and eating it. Try to keep your tongue away from the garlic, because the taste is very strong. Chase the garlic with a cup of peppermint tea (hot or chilled; you decide), which will help sweeten your digestive system after ingesting the pungent herb. As an alternative, enliven yourself with a snack of spicy hot pepper salsa and baked corn chips. The garlic and the salsa also help temporarily to clear sinus trouble and congestion from early autumn colds.

Herbal Baths—Hot baths comfort seasonal sore muscles and joints because floating in the water takes weight off stressed joints, and the heat helps relax tight areas. For extra relief, and to perfume the tub with relaxing aromas, pack about a quarter cup of dried chamomile or lavender in a large tea ball and hang it under the faucet so water flows through while the bath is running. A cup of Epsom salts added to the herb bath helps alleviate pain; a quarter cup of cider vinegar (herbed or not) will help alleviate itchy change-of-season skin, as will a half cup of baking soda. After your bath you may wish to rub on a topical herbal pain balm, such as one made from a compound of hot peppers, available at most pharmacies. Also note that stretching helps to dissipate lactic acid buildup in muscles, meaning that regular yoga, tai chi, and other such stretching movements may help to prevent and eventually eliminate pain.

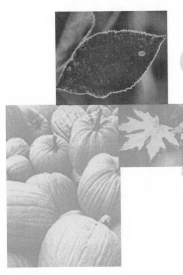

autumn:
the season
for storing

august, september, october

BEST TIME OF YEAR FOR:

✺ *Ripening your ideas and reaping the benefits*

✺ *Building on your strengths*

✺ *Nourishing yourself physically and mentally*

Keep a yang belly!" hollered Uncle Ho. And he waved good-bye as I sailed into Hong Kong bay on the Star Ferry one early autumn morning.

What Uncle Ho—my teacher, not really an uncle—meant by the odd farewell was that I should keep my digestion in good running order. He taught me that good health comes from nutritious foods and good digestion. If your digestion is off due to overconsumption of fats, sugars, junk food, alcohol, unmanaged stress, or certain medications, your body's ability to absorb nutrients will be diminished. When Uncle Ho advised me to "keep a yang belly," he meant that I should keep a digestive system that is warm and active—able to harvest the benefits from foods that the body needs for good health. This is especially important in autumn, when we reap the vitamins and minerals needed to keep us strong during the coming months.

Envision ancient tribes beneath an autumn sun, gathering and storing wholesome grains and vegetables to sustain themselves. Perhaps they learned the importance of autumn harvest from observing animals, who are instinctively aware of the food they eat. Even today in any city in autumn we can see squirrels storing nourishing nuts, and nonmigrating birds growing stout on seeds. Humans stocking up on autumn provisions are doing what sociologists call "gathering"—

THE MONTH OF AUGUST Our eighth month was named for Augustus Caesar, the first Roman emperor, and is thus thought of as the imperial or "crowned" month of the year during which chief food crops ripen for harvest and our eventual nourishment.

INTERESTING DATES IN AUGUST

August 23 (approximate)—The sun moves into the zodiac house of Virgo, symbolizing analytical powers. August (date floats)—Perseid Meteor Shower, where every ten to thirty seconds you can see a colorful meteor fly through the sky. Check your local paper for the exact date. August (date floats)—The harvest moon may arrive this month. This is the full moon that occurs before the autumnal equinox of about September 23. At this time the moon rises at nearly the same time the sun sets, and bright light floods the sky. The harvest moon was useful to farmers because it extended the workday with heavenly light. Weather permitting, this is a good evening for an al fresco meal.

a process (not unlike a squirrel with her nuts) of accumulation of goods that will fortify and strengthen the body.

Western science explains that this autumn gathering of nourishment has a positive effect on the immune system, a group of glands, organs, and body systems that work together to act as a weapon against infectious diseases, thus eliminating pathogens, toxins, and viruses from the body. A healthy immune system helps to strengthen the lungs and large intestines, toning them to combat autumn colds, coughs, and flu. Conversely, when the immune system is weak and the digestive system is not "a yang belly," we are unable to absorb nutrients. In addition, waste can build up and may result, for instance, in a head cold.

Along with wholesome foods, another way to enhance the immune system is through regular exercise, which helps improve circulation and eliminate immune-hampering toxins. Take a walk for twenty minutes four times a week; rent an exercise video and try it out; work out along with an exercise show on television; enroll in a yoga or tai chi class. Move your body regularly and it will serve you well.

Many experts also advise building immunities through regular meditation. Sitting quietly for five to twenty minutes once or twice a day helps to manage stress, which can disrupt the digestive system and render it unable to absorb sufficient nutrients. To try meditation, buy a relaxation tape and listen to at least five minutes of it once or twice a day. Or perform this meditation technique taught to me by a fourth grader. Sit in a chair in a quiet room, close your eyes, and slowly breathe in and out. As you do so, imagine a glow of light just beneath your navel that grows larger with each inhalation. Continue to breathe and glow until your whole body is filled with warm light. There is no correct number of breaths: However many it takes you is fine. When you're completely filled with the warm light, lift your arms over your head and exhale as if you were blowing out a candle. Experiment with this technique morning and evening. In addition, to keep a "yang belly," try one or more of these immune-building suggestions.

first aid kit for autumn

Stock up on these elixirs, potions, and ideas to prevent and soothe such autumn ills as coughs, colds, and flu.

Build Your Body—The roots and flower tops of the native American plant echinacea contain polysaccharide compounds that work at a cellular level to prevent viruses from invading the body. At the first sign of a cold or flu, begin to take the herb in tea, capsule, or tincture form. Echinacea is available at natural food stores and herb shops, and although it is always wise to check with a health professional before ingesting a new substance, experts recommend taking—for two weeks—one to three cups of tea per day; one to two capsules a day; or a teaspoon of tincture in a small amount of warm water three times a day.

To augment your echinacea therapy, the spicy, camphorus aroma of eucalyptus contains terpene compounds that are antiseptic against both local and airborne viruses. To put these qualities to use, combine twenty-five drops of essential oil of eucalyptus (available at pharmacies, natural food stores, and herb shops) and half a cup of distilled water in a spray bottle and mist the surfaces or air of your office, car, shared telephone, shared computer, pillow, or anywhere people close to you are sneezing or coughing. For a more personal defense, dot two drops of essential oil of eucalyptus on a cotton ball and tuck it into your bra or shirt pocket, inhaling the protective perfume throughout the day. To relieve upper respiratory congestion, dot two drops on a tissue and inhale for two to three minutes; or put five drops in a bowl of warm water, lean over the bowl, tent a towel over your head, and inhale the soothing vapors for about five minutes. To ingest the healing powers of eucalyptus, drop a menthol-eucalyptus cough lozenge (available at pharmacies) in a cup of water. Add a tablespoon of lemon juice, then microwave on full power until the lozenge has dissolved, about four minutes. If you don't have a microwave, boil the lozenge, lemon juice, and water in a small saucepan for about four minutes.

Another spicy, clean-smelling essence is tea-tree (or Ti-tree). It's an

THE MONTH OF SEPTEMBER
The name of our ninth month comes from the Latin "seven," because it was the seventh month in the old Roman year. September is known throughout the world as the "harvest month," a time to reap and gather what you need. In literature, to be "Septembered" is to be "warmed by autumnal tints."

INTERESTING DATES IN SEPTEMBER
September 7—*Festival of Durga*, in India, marking a five-day celebration that encourages the settling of spats and the reuniting of people. On the fifth day, a symbol of the argument is flung into a flowing river, to forever let go of the grievance.

MORE INTERESTING DATES
IN SEPTEMBER
*September 15—Birthday of
the Moon,* in China,
honoring all that is lunar
and feminine. Recently
harvested fruits are feasted
upon, and people go out at
night to bathe in cool
moonlight. *September* (date
floats)—Check your local
paper for the exact date of
the Harvest Moon, the full
moon that occurs right
before the autumnal
equinox. On this evening
the moon rises at about
the same time the sun
sets, illuminating our late-
day activities with celestial
light. *September 23*
(approximately)—*The
Autumnal Equinox,* marking
the time when the hours of
daylight and darkness are
equal. On this day, the sun
enters the zodiac sign of
Libra, whose icon is a set
of scales, symbolizing
equality and balance.

antiseptic and anti-infective to respiratory diseases. Use the essential oil (available at pharmacies, natural food stores, and herb shops) in a mist, as for the eucalyptus above. Or make a protective lotion by combining seven to ten drops of the essence in a quarter cup of your favorite body lotion and rubbing it on your upper arms, neck, and chest before venturing out. You can also take a tea-tree bath to replenish your strength by adding seven drops of essence to the warm water. Soak for about twenty minutes in the evening, after a cold, damp, autumn day.

In addition, vitamin C helps strengthen immunities and guard against infective diseases by increasing the body's production of protective T-cells and interferon. One way to take vitamin C is in the form of the Indian Ayurvedic jam, chavanprash, available at natural food stores and Indian markets. Chavanprash is made from the amla fruit, each of which contains about 3,000 milligrams of easily absorbable vitamin C. In chavanprash the amlas are mixed with other immune-supporting herbs and cooked down to make a thick paste. Experts recommend one teaspoon twice a day, swirled into tea, spread on toast, or just taken off the spoon. Note that overconsumption of alcohol, and frequent ingestion of aspirin, may deplete the body's levels of vitamin C, a critical autumn nutrient.

In addition to these herbs and nutrients, many experts advise taking a full spectrum pro-biotic, or acidophilus-type supplement, to encourage the abundance of beneficial intestinal flora. Excess coffee and alcohol consumption, as well as antibiotics and some other medications, can deplete these flora, which can lead to poor absorption of nutrients and impaired immunities.

Build Your Mind—A study at Southern Methodist University showed that keeping a "stress diary," or making notes about tense moments and events, can help build immunities. Participants in the study wrote for about twenty minutes a day, about fears, anxieties, anger, and sadness, both past and present. This helped them identify and release "toxic thoughts" that could eventually lead to lowered immunities.

Build Your Herbal Pantry—Be sure to keep oregano on hand, since its peppery volatile oils can help abate the symptoms of autumn colds and indigestion. Combine a tablespoon each of dried oregano (or two tablespoons fresh) and fennel seeds with vinegar and a splash of olive oil to use as a marinade for grilled fish or vegetables. Or, to soothe the sniffles, sprinkle a tablespoon of dried oregano in a bowl of hot water and inhale the comforting vapors.

Spicy cinnamon, both stick and ground, is used by herbalists to treat autumn chills. Its volatile oils help increase circulation, especially in the upper respiratory area. To try it, make a medicinal wine: In a covered glass jar, add three cinnamon sticks to two cups of dry red wine and steep for two weeks. Keep the jar in a sunny window, shaking it daily. Sip up to a quarter cup of the mixture in the evenings, to warm you on a frosty night. If you don't drink alcohol, add the cinnamon sticks to apple juice and let the mixture steep for the same amount of time as for wine, in the refrigerator, heating as needed before sipping.

THE MONTH OF OCTOBER
The name of our tenth month comes from the Latin for "eight," marking the eighth month in the old Roman year. In many cultures, October is a time of harvest celebrations, such as Oktoberfest in Germany. October is often called the "ale-brewing" month, because of the hops harvest.

INTERESTING DATES IN OCTOBER

October 13—Festival of the Floating Lamps, in Thailand, honoring Buddha, who is said to have walked upon the riverbanks in that country. Lanterns are lighted and set adrift in the rivers to please Buddha and to lead others along their spiritual way. *October 22* (approximate)—The sun moves into the zodiac sign of Scorpio, symbolizing strength and transformation.

strengthening
autumn beverages

Open your kitchen cabinet and you're sure to find at least one herb or spice that can serve as a healing autumn tea. Dried marjoram from the supermarket—one teaspoon steeped in one cup of just-boiled water for five minutes—makes a soothing digestive tonic. Try dillweed for the same purpose. Add a pinch of ground cinnamon to your morning coffee or tea to increase circulation and energy. You may also wish to stock up on the ingredients for one or more of these bolstering autumn beverages.

green tea

To manufacture this tea, camellia leaves are harvested from the plant, then lightly steamed and sometimes rolled. If you've had a pale greenish tea that's mild and slightly fruity in a Chinese or Japanese restaurant, you've had green tea. This common beverage contains polysaccharide compounds that help strengthen the immune system, and there is no better time to imbibe these benefits than in the fall.

1 teaspoon green tea, or 1 tea bag   1 cup just-boiled water

Combine the tea and water in a ceramic mug, cover, and let the liquid steep for 30 seconds to 2 minutes. Then discard the leaves and sip up to 3 cups a day.

MAKES ONE SERVING; ABOUT 2 CALORIES; NO ADDED FAT.

VARIATIONS:

Try a type of green tea called genmai-cha (cha *means "tea"*) containing roasted brown rice as well as tea, available at natural food stores and Asian markets. The rice gives the brewed tea a warm and nutty flavor, and Japanese folklore holds that the tea helps to strengthen immunities by acting as a lymphatic tonic.

Green tea scented with orange or jasmine blossoms is a pleasant restorative with fortifying benefits you need this time of year. Find either floral version at Asian markets or tea shops.

Try a tea called kukicha, made from roasted camellia twigs, rather than leaves. It's available at natural food stores and Asian markets in bulk and tea bag forms. Follow brewing instructions on the box, which should be to steep the bags and boil the bulk twigs. Kukicha tea is offered in Japan as a soothing digestive tonic. Make extra to bring to work for a midafternoon restorative teatime. If you are feeling dehydrated, mix half a portion of brewed kukicha with an equal amount of apple juice and drink warmed or chilled.

If the weather is damp: Add a slice of fresh gingerroot during steeping.

If the weather is dry: Add a slice of dried Chinese licorice root or a slice of fresh orange during steeping. Or, to make an iced version, double the amount of tea and add ice after steeping.

shiitake broth with ginger

If the weather is damp: Increase the gingerroot to 2 slices and garnish with minced scallion.

If the weather is dry: Garnish with lemon zest before serving.

Shiitake mushrooms, available dried at Asian markets, natural food stores, and many supermarkets, contain polysaccharide compounds that help nourish the immune system.

2 dried shiitake mushrooms
1 slice fresh gingerroot

2 cups just-boiled water or kukicha tea (page 233)

In a small teapot, soak the mushrooms and gingerroot in the water, covered, for 1 hour. Then drain, reheat, and sip. As an option, thinly slice the mushroom caps (discard tough stems) and add to the broth. You may also use the broth as a soup stock or base for sauces.

MAKES TWO 1-CUP SERVINGS; 3 TO 5 CALORIES PER CUP; NO ADDED FAT.

rosemary and lavender tisane

If the weather is damp: Add a bay leaf to the tisane while steeping.

If the weather is dry: Add a dried rose petal or I drop of rosewater to the steeping tea.

"Tisane" is a French term for an herbal tea or infusion that produces a pleasantly mild medicinal effect in those who drink it. In the case of this brew, the rosemary warms a chilled autumn body by increasing circulation; and the lavender serves as a mild nervine and digestive tonic.

1 teaspoon dried rosemary
1 teaspoon dried lavender

1 cup just-boiled water

Steep the rosemary and lavender in the water, covered, for 5 minutes. Then discard the herbs and sip the tea.

MAKES ONE SERVING; 2 CALORIES; NO ADDED FAT.

autumn immuno-tea i

Drinking this flavorful brew can help prevent autumn colds and flu. The ginger-root warms the body by stimulating circulation; the echinacea helps stop invading viruses at a cellular level; and the raspberry leaf helps tone the intestines so excess waste is properly eliminated from the body.

1 teaspoon finely shredded dried
   echinacea root

1 teaspoon dried raspberry leaf

2 slices fresh gingerroot

2 cups just-boiled water

If the weather is damp: Increase the gingerroot to 3 slices.

If the weather is dry: Add 5 raisins to the tea during steeping.

Combine all of the ingredients in a nonmetallic container and steep, covered, for 5 minutes. If the echinacea is not finely shredded, steep it by itself for 5 minutes before adding the raspberry leaf and gingerroot. Discard the herbs and sip. Two cups a day is recommended.

MAKES TWO 1-CUP SERVINGS; 2 CALORIES PER SERVING; NO ADDED FAT.

autumn immuno-tea ii

These herbs come from China, where studies show that the schizandra has particular ability in building resistance to disease. Find these berries at herb shops, natural food stores, and Asian markets.

2 tablespoons dried schizandra berry

2 tablespoons dried lycii berry

1 slice dried Chinese licorice root

3 cups water

If the weather is damp: Add a slice of fresh gingerroot when simmering.

If the weather is dry: Double the licorice root.

Soak the schizandra berries in water to cover, overnight. Don't skip this step, since it removes excess tannin from the berries, which when left in may cause constipation. Drain the water and rinse the berries. Then combine them in a small saucepan along with the lycii berry, licorice root, and the fresh water. Gently simmer the decoction for about 15 minutes, then discard the herbs and sip half the amount (about 1¼ cups) a day. If you have high blood pressure, eliminate the licorice root, as it may aggravate the condition.

MAKES ABOUT 2½ CUPS OR 2 SERVINGS; ABOUT 10 CALORIES PER SERVING; NO ADDED FAT.

carotene cocktail

If the weather is damp: Swirl in a pinch of ground cinnamon before drinking.

———

If the weather is dry: Add a dried apricot to the juices while heating to a boil. Keep the apricot in while steeping the chamomile, then discard or enjoy the apricot as a snack.

Should you suffer from upper respiratory congestion, the beta carotene in this aromatic elixir can help deter mucus production.

½ cup carrot juice

½ cup apple juice

1 teaspoon dried chamomile

In a small saucepan, heat the carrot and apple juices until just boiling. Pour them into a large mug to which you've added the chamomile. Cover and steep for about 4 minutes. Then discard the chamomile and sip as needed.

MAKES ONE SERVING; 80 CALORIES; NO ADDED FAT.

breathe-better tea i

If the weather is damp: Add ½ teaspoon dried yarrow.

———

If the weather is dry: Add ½ teaspoon dried catnip.

If you have a cold, the sage in this infusion will help to calm inflamed upper respiratory membranes, allowing you to breathe more freely. The hyssop is what herbalists call an "antispasmodic," soothing irritated bronchials and lungs. The tea as a whole is a "diaphoretic," a substance that, when ingested, helps relieve feverish conditions.

1 teaspoon dried sage

1 teaspoon dried hyssop

1 slice fresh lemon

1 cup just-boiled water

In a large mug, combine all of the ingredients and let the tea steep, covered, for 5 minutes. Discard the solids and sip the tea as needed.

MAKES ONE SERVING; 2 CALORIES; NO ADDED FAT.

breathe-better tea ii

This is a variation of the classic North American elixir for autumn colds and sinus congestion. Thyme has been added because it contains an anti-infective compound called thymol.

If the weather is damp:
Double the thyme.

If the weather is dry:
Double the peppermint.

1 teaspoon dried peppermint

1 teaspoon dried elder flower
   (available at natural food stores)

1 teaspoon dried thyme

1 cup just-boiled water

In a large mug, combine all of the ingredients and steep, covered, for 5 minutes. Discard the solids and sip the tea as needed.

MAKES ONE SERVING; 2 CALORIES; NO ADDED FAT.

breathe-better tea iii

Mullein, the main ingredient in this tonic, contains mucilage, gums, and immune-enhancing saponins that work together to help heal an autumn cough.

If the weather is damp:
Double the mullein.

If the weather is dry:
Double the mint.

1 teaspoon dried mullein (available
   at natural food stores)

1 teaspoon dried mint

1 slice fresh lemon

1 cup just-boiled water

Combine all of the ingredients in a large mug and steep, covered, for about 8 minutes. Discard the plant material and sip one to three cups a day.

MAKES ONE SERVING; 3 CALORIES; NO ADDED FAT.

breathe-better tea iv

If the weather is damp:
Add a splash of hot pepper
sauce before drinking.

If the weather is dry: Add
a splash of lemon juice
before drinking.

This vegetable-based brew is a popular folk cure in Japan, where it soothes symptoms of head colds, as well as scratchy coughs. One way it may work is that it contains spicy radish, which helps clear clogged respiratory passages.

2 tablespoons coarsely grated carrot
2 tablespoons coarsely grated daikon
   radish or other radish

Splash of regular or reduced-sodium
   soy sauce
1 cup just-boiled water

In a large mug, combine the carrot, radish, and soy sauce. Pour on the water and drink hot. When you're finished, eat the grated vegetables.

MAKES ONE SERVING; 35 CALORIES; NO ADDED FAT.

strengthening autumn foods

Although it may seem natural to "bulk up" at this time of year as a defense against the impending cold, it is best to eat lightly but well to "keep a yang belly." Eat slowly so your stomach can tell when it's not quite full, Uncle Ho advised, noting that it takes several minutes for the brain to become alerted to the fact that the stomach is full. Overeating (as well as abundant fat, sugar, white flour, and alcohol in the diet) can cause the digestive system to become overtaxed, and thus unable to efficiently eliminate toxins. These unwanted accumulations can appear as autumn colds, coughs, and flu—the body's way of ridding itself of excesses.

Nutrient-rich harvest foods are the wise and healthful choice, including broccoli, cauliflower, cabbage, garlic, onions, autumn greens, winter squash, peppers, and fall fruits. But remember, if you feel at all "under the weather," it's best to drink a strengthening tea, avoiding food until your "yang belly" returns.

broccoli
the helpful head

One sure way to judge a good nutritionist is by how he or she looks. If she's vibrant and fit, she probably knows what she's talking about. That's how I came to heed the advice of a nutritionist I call "Mr. Broccoli": He looked well, was energetic, and said that one of his secrets was eating broccoli every day.

Not a bad idea, since broccoli contains immune-enhancing vitamin C and beta carotene; folate, potassium, calcium, and B_6 for steady nerves; chlorophyll for good digestion; and only 22 calories in each half cup of cooked vegetable. In addition, broccoli contains cancer-fighting compounds called "indoles."

buying broccoli

Choose firm heads that are vivid green or purplish and free of yellow spots. The fresher the broccoli, the more vitamin C it will offer you. At home, use a sharp paring knife to poke a few air holes in the produce bag, then refrigerate for up to five days.

> ### quick cooking tip for broccoli
> Steam broccoli florets until just tender and bright green, about five minutes. Then toss with fresh lemon juice, olive oil, and a pinch of sea salt. Serve warm or at room temperature as a side dish, or tossed with hot pasta or rice.

broccoli soup with potato and leek

In addition to the nourishing broccoli, this soup contains leek, shallots, and garlic, offering extra body-guard compounds to ward off autumn colds and flu.

1 tablespoon olive oil
¾ pound broccoli, chopped
1 large potato, chopped
1 leek, chopped
2 shallots, chopped
1 clove garlic, minced
2 cups vegetable stock or water
1 teaspoon minced fresh thyme, or
  ½ teaspoon dried

1 teaspoon minced fresh oregano, or
  ½ teaspoon dried
2 teaspoons prepared mustard
1 cup nonfat soy or skim milk
¼ cup crumbled feta cheese or
  grated soy mozzarella
Pinch of sea salt

If the weather is damp: Add freshly ground black pepper when adding the salt.

If the weather is dry: Garnish with chopped fresh tomatoes before serving.

Heat a large stockpot, and add the oil. Sauté the broccoli, potato, leek, shallots, and garlic, over medium-high heat, stirring frequently, for about 5 minutes.

Add 1 cup of the stock or water, along with the thyme and oregano, then cover loosely and simmer until the vegetables are very tender, about 20 minutes. Stir occasionally.

Let the soup cool, then pour it into a food processor or blender along with the mustard and process until just smooth. Don't overprocess or the potato will become gummy.

Pour the puree back into the pot and add the remaining stock, milk, cheese, and salt, and heat gently, stirring well, until the cheese is warm. Serve warm as a side dish for lunch or dinner.

MAKES FOUR SERVINGS; 171 CALORIES PER SERVING; 5 GRAMS OF FAT; 27 PERCENT OF CALORIES FROM FAT.

autumn vegetable pâté

If the weather is damp: Top with spicy salsa or spicy mustard.

———

If the weather is dry: Serve with a crisp green salad.

With this flavorful dish you can reap the body-bolstering benefits of the seasonal harvest—vitamin C, beta carotene, and calcium.

2 cups chopped broccoli

1 cup chopped cauliflower

1 cup sliced carrots

¼ cup good-quality tomato salsa

½ cup rolled oats

2 tablespoons cornmeal

¼ cup bread crumbs

4 egg whites, or ½ cup commercial egg substitute

1 tablespoon minced fresh thyme, or 1½ teaspoons dried

¼ cup part-skim mozzarella or nonfat soy mozzarella

Preheat the oven to 400°F. Lightly oil a loaf pan.

Blanch the broccoli, cauliflower, and carrots in boiling water until just tender, about 5 minutes. Or microwave them on full power for about 5 minutes. Drain and pat dry. In a medium bowl, combine the blanched vegetables with the remaining ingredients.

Press the vegetable mixture firmly into the prepared loaf pan with your hands, smoothing out the top. Bake until firm, 20 to 25 minutes. Let the pâté cool slightly, then slice into 4 pieces and serve warm or slightly chilled as an appetizer, entrée, or packed as a savory office lunch.

MAKES 4 SERVINGS; 135 CALORIES PER SERVING; TRACE OF FAT.

broccoli with fresh tomatoes and lemon vinaigrette

This salad, which takes less than 10 minutes to make, is an easy way to garner the fortifying properties of broccoli. What's more, the oregano serves as an autumn digestive tonic.

1 pound broccoli, cut into bite-sized
  pieces
2 ripe medium tomatoes, chopped
Juice of 1 lemon
2 teaspoons olive oil

Pinch of dry mustard
2 teaspoons minced fresh oregano,
  or 1 teaspoon dried
Pinch of sea salt

If the weather is damp: Add a splash of hot pepper sauce to the lemon mixture.

If the weather is dry: Serve with lemon wedges for squeezing.

Steam the broccoli over boiling water until the broccoli is bright green and just tender, about 5 minutes.

Meanwhile, tip the tomatoes into a serving bowl, adding the broccoli when it's ready.

In a small bowl, whisk together the lemon juice, oil, mustard, oregano, and salt. Pour over the broccoli mixture and toss gently to combine. Serve warm or at room temperature as a lunch or dinner salad, first course, or side dish.

MAKES 4 SERVINGS; 90 CALORIES PER SERVING; 2 GRAMS OF FAT; 20 PERCENT OF CALORIES FROM FAT.

chinese-style noodle cakes

If the weather is damp: Add a minced fresh jalapeño before baking.

If the weather is dry: Serve with a salad of crisp greens.

This is called "Two Sides Brown" in China, where it is enjoyed as a warming breakfast, lunch, and autumn snack at any season. The garlic, scallions, and gingerroot help increase circulation, thus taking the edge off the chill outside.

1 cup steamed, chopped broccoli
1 shallot, minced
1 clove garlic, minced
2 scallions, minced
½ teaspoon finely grated fresh
    gingerroot

1 teaspoon toasted (dark) sesame oil
3 cups cooked spaghetti
2 egg whites, or ¼ cup commercial
    egg substitute
Pinch of sea salt

In a large bowl, combine all of the ingredients. Using your hands, work the mixture so that it's moist all over and so that the broccoli is well distributed throughout.

Spray a 10-inch nonstick sauté pan with nonstick spray and add the noodle mixture. Pat it down into a pancake, set a 10-inch plate atop it, and weight the plate with a full teakettle or other similarly heavy object. Let the noodle cake cook over medium heat for about 10 minutes.

To flip the noodle cake, remove the weight, then pick up the skillet in one hand and hold the plate securely in the other. Reverse positions so that the plate is on the bottom and the skillet (upside down) is on top. Put the skillet back on the burner and, with the plate right next to it, slide the noodle cake right in. Set the plate and weight on top and bake for 10 minutes more, taking care not to burn the broccoli.

When the noodle cake is ready, slide it onto a plate, cut it into wedges with kitchen shears, and serve warm for brunch, lunch, or dinner. The wedges reheat well, so pack one to take to work for lunch.

MAKES 4 SERVINGS; 190 CALORIES PER SERVING; 1 GRAM OF FAT; 5 PERCENT OF CALORIES FROM FAT.

broccoli lo mein

This easy stir-fry, made with vegetables and noodles, contains virus-fighting beta carotene. In fact, just one serving offers over twice the Recommended Daily Allowance (RDA) for the vitamin. Though the ingredients list looks long, it's an easy and quick recipe for busy weekday nights.

3 cups cooked spaghetti

¼ cup vegetable stock

1 tablespoon regular or reduced-sodium soy sauce

1 tablespoon balsamic vinegar

1 tablespoon cornstarch

1 clove garlic, minced

½ teaspoon finely grated fresh gingerroot

4 teaspoons canola oil

2 shallots, sliced

2 carrots, julienned

1 red bell pepper, julienned

1 cup broccoli florets

¼ teaspoon toasted (dark) sesame oil

2 scallions, minced

If the weather is damp: Increase the gingerroot to 1 teaspoon.

If the weather is dry: Serve with warm or iced mint tea.

Refrigerate the cooked pasta for at least 10 minutes to avoid later clumping.

In a small bowl, whisk together the stock, soy sauce, vinegar, cornstarch, garlic, and gingerroot. Set aside.

Heat a wok or large sauté pan on medium-high. Add 1 teaspoon of the canola oil and heat. Add the spaghetti and sauté until it's lightly browned, about 2 minutes. Remove the spaghetti from the pan and set aside.

Add the remaining 3 teaspoons of canola oil to the pan and heat for about 1 minute. Add the shallots, carrots, red pepper, and broccoli and sauté until fragrant and just beginning to soften and brown, about 4 minutes. Pour the sauce over the vegetables and stir until thickened and shiny, about 2 minutes. Add the spaghetti, sesame oil, and scallions, toss to combine, and serve as a lunch or dinner entrée.

MAKES 4 SERVINGS; 195 CALORIES PER SERVING; 6 GRAMS OF FAT; 28 PERCENT OF CALORIES FROM FAT.

cauliflower
no pale cousin

I was pleased to learn from an Ayurvedic Indian doctor that a cup of cauliflower, despite its mild and pale appearance, contains nearly 100 percent of the Recommended Daily Allowance (RDA) for infection-fighting vitamin C. Because of this, it is especially recommended to vegetarians in India who rely on dried beans as a source of iron, since vitamin C enhances absorption of the fatigue-fighting mineral. And since it is low in calories—22 per cup—and contains virtually no fat, cauliflower is a dieter's dream. The Ayurvedic doctor also shared a secret for making cauliflower easy to digest: For each head, add a teaspoon of whole mustard seeds to the cooking water or sauce.

the hard truth

Hard cooking water can make your cauliflower turn yellow. To prevent the problem, add one teaspoon of lemon juice to the boiling or blanching water before cooking.

mustard-roasted cauliflower

In addition to creating a more digestible dish, the mustard contains magnesium, a mineral important in fighting fall fatigue. The garlic helps, too, by increasing circulation.

1 whole cauliflower
¼ cup prepared mustard
2 cloves garlic, finely minced

1 teaspoon minced fresh dillweed, or
½ teaspoon dried

Preheat the oven to 400°F.

Remove the leaves from the cauliflower. In a small dish, combine the mustard, garlic, and dillweed, and spread the mixture over the entire head of cauliflower. Set the cauliflower, stem down, in a ring mold and roast until fragrant, browned, and tender, about 1 hour. Slice the florets from the stem and serve warm as a lunch or dinner side dish.

MAKES 4 SMALL SERVINGS; 26 CALORIES PER SERVING; NO ADDED FAT.

If the weather is damp: Add ½ teaspoon hot pepper sauce (or to taste) to the mustard mixture before spreading it on.

If the weather is dry: Garnish the roasted cauliflower with minced fresh cilantro.

braised cauliflower with mustard sauce

If the weather is damp:
Add a dried hot pepper to
the stock when simmering.

If the weather is dry:
Instead of 1½ cups stock,
use 1 cup stock and
½ cup tomato juice.

The clovelike scent of bay adds a refreshing top note to this dish, as well as soothing digestive qualities.

1½ cups vegetable stock or water
1 teaspoon mustard seeds
3 bay leaves
1 pound cauliflower, cut into
   bite-sized pieces

1 tablespoon prepared mustard
Pinch of sea salt
Minced fresh dillweed or parsley for
   garnish

In a large skillet, combine the stock or water, mustard seeds, and bay leaves and bring to a boil. Add the cauliflower and simmer, loosely covered, until tender, about 8 minutes.

Remove the cauliflower from the stock and arrange it in a serving dish. Strain the stock and put it back in the skillet, bringing to a boil. When the stock has been reduced to about ¼ cup, whisk in the mustard and salt and pour over the cauliflower. Sprinkle with the dillweed and serve warm as a lunch or dinner side dish.

MAKES 4 SERVINGS; 21 CALORIES PER SERVING; NO ADDED FAT.

cauliflower with ginger

Herbalists say that gingerroot aids digestibility of such vegetables as cauliflower. In addition, gingerroot warms the body, promoting a "yang belly."

1 teaspoon olive oil

1 teaspoon cuminseed

2 tablespoons finely grated fresh gingerroot

1 head cauliflower, cut into florets

¼ cup vegetable stock or water

Juice of ½ lemon

Hot pepper sauce to taste

Minced fresh cilantro for garnish

If the weather is damp: Substitute 2 minced scallions for the cilantro.

If the weather is dry: Be generous with the cilantro.

Heat a large sauté pan on medium-high, and add the oil. Sauté the cuminseed until they are fragrant, about 1 minute. Add the gingerroot, cauliflower, stock or water, lemon, and hot pepper sauce, stirring well. Reduce the heat to medium, cover loosely, and let simmer until the cauliflower is almost tender, about 5 minutes. Remove the cover, increase the heat to high, and stir constantly until all of the liquid has been absorbed and the cauliflower is tender, about 2 minutes more. If you need more liquid to do this, just add more stock or water. Sprinkle with the cilantro before serving warm as a lunch or dinner side dish.

MAKES 4 SERVINGS; 35 CALORIES PER SERVING; 1 GRAM OF FAT; 27 PERCENT OF CALORIES FROM FAT.

cabbage
the cure-all

In what was once East Germany, I lunched on a Greek salad complete with olives and feta cheese, and topped with sauerkraut. I was not really surprised, as I had noticed throughout Germany that cabbage, both fresh and fermented, was added to everything—rice, scrambled eggs, chicken casseroles, even tomato sauce. I later learned that ever since the Germans conquered Rome, where they discovered cabbage, they have held the vegetable in high esteem. Many Germans claim that cabbage, eaten regularly, can relieve asthma, purify the blood, cure constipation, prevent sciatica, and lengthen life.

Science, too, praises cabbage for the indole compounds this vegetable contains which help prevent cancer. What's more, cabbage is a good source of immune-boosting vitamin C and digestion-toning fiber. One cup of shredded raw cabbage contains 16 calories and virtually no fat. Use it in place of some of the lettuce in a green salad and experience what the Germans have known for centuries.

cabbage lore

Cabbage is the September 19 birthday flower, symbolizing profit and good luck in business. Throughout history, cabbage has been a badge of those who are independent and self-willed.

hot and sour soup

Chinese healers say that hot (spicy) foods help increase circulation, especially in chilly weather; and that sour foods are an important tonic for the liver, an organ that is critical to all body functions, especially digestion.

If the weather is damp: Be liberal with the hot pepper sauce and black pepper.

4 cups vegetable stock
2½ cups finely shredded cabbage
¼ cup finely shredded bamboo shoots
1 tablespoon regular or reduced-sodium soy sauce
1 teaspoon finely grated fresh gingerroot
3 cloves garlic, minced

2 tablespoons rice or white vinegar
2 tablespoons cornstarch mixed with ¼ cup water
1 teaspoon toasted (dark) sesame oil
1 tablespoon hot pepper sauce, or to taste
Freshly ground black pepper to taste
3 tablespoons minced fresh chives or Chinese chives

If the weather is dry: Substitute sliced water chestnuts for the bamboo shoots.

In a large soup pot, combine the stock, cabbage, bamboo shoots, soy sauce, gingerroot, garlic, and vinegar and bring to a boil. Reduce the heat to low, cover loosely, and simmer until the cabbage has wilted, about 4 minutes. Stir the cornstarch mixture and pour it into the soup, stirring until it has slightly thickened. Add the sesame oil, hot pepper sauce, black pepper, and chives, and serve warm for lunch or dinner.

MAKES 4 SERVINGS; 70 CALORIES PER SERVING; 1 GRAM OF FAT; 13 PERCENT OF CALORIES FROM FAT.

sautéed cabbage with toasted fennel seeds

*If the weather is damp:
Add a minced fresh
jalapeño when sautéing.*

*If the weather is dry: Use
tomato juice instead of
vegetable stock.*

Fennel seeds contain aromatic compounds that soothe digestion—especially important with such sulfur-containing vegetables as cabbage.

1 tablespoon fennel seeds	4 cups shredded cabbage
1 teaspoon olive oil	2 scallions, minced
⅓ cup vegetable stock or water	2 tablespoons freshly grated
2 cloves garlic, minced	Parmesan cheese or soy Parmesan

Heat a large dry sauté pan on medium-high and add the fennel seeds. Stir until the fennel seeds are lightly browned and fragrant, about 2 minutes. Remove them from the pan and set them aside.

In the same hot pan, add the olive oil, stock or water, garlic, and cabbage, and sauté until the cabbage is cooked through but still crunchy, about 5 minutes. Tip the cabbage into a large serving bowl along with the scallions, fennel seeds, and Parmesan, and serve warm as a lunch or dinner side dish.

MAKES 4 SERVINGS; 65 CALORIES PER SERVING; 1.5 GRAMS OF FAT; 20 PERCENT OF CALORIES FROM FAT.

cabbage salad with sesame and ginger

Gingerroot, such as that which flavors this savory slaw, contains volatile oils that act as a digestive stimulant.

5 cups finely shredded cabbage

2 carrots, coarsely grated

3 scallions, minced

¼ cup lemon juice

1 tablespoon toasted (dark)
  sesame oil

1 clove garlic, minced

½ teaspoon finely grated fresh
  gingerroot

1 tablespoon sesame seeds

*If the weather is damp:
Increase the garlic to
2 cloves and serve at
room temperature.*

*If the weather is dry: Serve
with lemon wedges for
squeezing.*

In a large bowl, combine the cabbage, carrots, and scallions. In a small bowl, whisk together the lemon juice, sesame oil, garlic, and gingerroot. Pour over the cabbage and toss well to combine.

Tip the sesame seeds into a dry sauté pan and heat on medium-high, stirring well, until they're lightly toasted and fragrant, about 1 minute. Transfer to a mortar or spice grinder and crush but don't make a paste. Sprinkle over the salad and serve at room temperature or very slightly chilled for lunch or dinner.

MAKES 4 SERVINGS; 75 CALORIES PER SERVING; 2.5 GRAMS OF FAT; 30 PERCENT OF CALORIES FROM FAT.

red cabbage salad with creamy chive dressing

If the weather is damp: Increase the garlic to 2 cloves.

If the weather is dry: Serve with lime wedges for squeezing.

Chives, garlic, and scallions all contribute sulfur compounds to help stave off autumn ills.

3 cups finely shredded red cabbage
2 cups finely shredded white or
    green cabbage
1 carrot, coarsely grated
3 scallions, minced
¼ cup lime juice

¼ cup plain nonfat yogurt or soy
    yogurt
1 clove garlic, minced
½ teaspoon finely grated fresh
    gingerroot
2 tablespoons minced fresh chives

In a medium bowl, combine the cabbages, carrot, and scallions. In a small bowl, whisk together the lime juice, yogurt, garlic, and gingerroot. Scoop over the cabbage and toss well to combine. Sprinkle with the chives and serve at room temperature or very slightly chilled for lunch or dinner.

MAKES 4 SERVINGS; 60 CALORIES PER SERVING; 1 GRAM OF FAT; 15 PERCENT OF CALORIES FROM FAT.

marinated brussels sprouts

Russian and Ayurvedic herbalists hold that dillweed helps soothe and tone digestion—specially important with these gas-inducing tiny cabbages.

10 ounces Brussels sprouts

1 bay leaf

2 carrots, peeled and julienned

Juice of 1 lemon

1 teaspoon balsamic vinegar

2 teaspoons olive oil

1 teaspoon minced fresh dillweed, or
   ½ teaspoon dried

½ teaspoon dillseed

½ teaspoon celery seed

1 clove garlic, very finely minced

Freshly ground black pepper to taste

Pinch of sea salt

If the weather is damp: Increase the garlic to 2 cloves.

If the weather is dry: Serve on a nest of curly red lettuce.

Clean and trim the Brussels sprouts, then carve an X in the bottom of each. Add the sprouts and bay leaf to a pot of boiling water and loosely cover. The water should just cover the sprouts. Simmer until the sprouts are bright green and tender, 9 to 10 minutes, adding the carrots for the last minute of cooking.

Meanwhile, in a medium bowl, combine the remaining ingredients. When the sprouts and carrots are ready, drain and pat them dry and add to the marinade, letting them marinate refrigerated for at least an hour. Serve at room temperature with lunch or dinner.

MAKES 4 SERVINGS; 90 CALORIES PER SERVING; 2 GRAMS OF FAT; 20 PERCENT OF CALORIES FROM FAT.

garlic and onions
bulbs for the body

"First we 'kill' the onion," said my Israeli dinner guest, as he volunteered to make the salad, which began with two pounds of raw yellow onions. He peeled and thinly sliced the pungent bulbs, then plunged them into a huge pot of lightly salted water for about thirty seconds. Once they were drained and patted dry, he tossed the onions with olive oil, lemon juice, sea salt, and freshly ground pepper, then chilled the salad for about twenty minutes. The blanching "killed" the harsh onion bite, he claimed, leaving them sweet and crisp. And indeed it did.

Garlic, too, can be "killed" before cooking, if its properties when eaten raw are abusive to your digestion. This problem tends to occur more in hot weather, which accentuates garlic's hot and spicy effects on your body. In fact, those warming effects are coveted and more easily digested in the chillier autumn. But if you need to eliminate the "heat" in any season, peel as many cloves as you require and boil for at least thirty seconds before adding to sauces, salad dressings, or whatever you're preparing. For pasta, simply add the garlic to the boiling water the last minute or two of cooking, then drain and remove, crush, and add to the sauce.

The volatile oils that give garlic and onions their characteristic taste and aroma are sulfur compounds which help protect the body from viral infections and act as a digestive tonic. As an autumn elixir you may wish to eat one clove of garlic, or half a small onion a day. Taken raw, garlic and onion contain more of the coveted sulfur compounds, but you can double your daily amount if you choose to eat them cooked in such bean, grain, and vegetable dishes as are offered here.

The onion has long been a spiritual symbol of unity, suggested perhaps by its many layers comprising a greater whole. In some African countries, to dream of an onion is good luck. This belief may have prompted people to carry onions in their pockets to ward off disease. Similarly, garlic has been used as a talisman against plague. In one French tale, thieves who, during the plague, robbed the pockets of the dead kept healthy by drinking and rubbing themselves with garlic-steeped vinegar.

quick cooking tip for garlic and onion

To deepen the flavor of soups and stews, add one onion and one or two cloves of garlic for every four servings. The longer they're cooked, the sweeter and less pungent onion and garlic become, which is what chefs call "working the onion." For instance, sautéing onion and garlic long and slow before adding them to a dish will produce a rich and deeply sweet taste, whereas tossing them raw into the pot will give the dish a sharper, hotter flavor.

spicy chick-pea soup with peanuts

If the weather is damp: Sprinkle with freshly ground pepper before serving.

———

If the weather is dry: Double the amount of cilantro.

This easy-to-prepare soup contains garlic and onion, as well as chick-peas, which provide a good dose of immune-boosting folate.

1½ cups dried chick-peas
1 tablespoon olive oil
3 cloves garlic, minced
1 large onion, minced
6 cups vegetable stock or water
2 tablespoons regular or reduced-sodium soy sauce

1 tablespoon hot pepper sauce, or to taste
¼ cup chopped peanuts
¼ cup minced fresh cilantro or parsley

Soak the chick-peas in water to cover overnight. Then drain.

In a large soup pot heat the oil on medium-high. Add the garlic and onion and sauté until they're fragrant and just tender, about 4 minutes. Add the soaked chick-peas, the vegetable stock or water, soy sauce, and hot pepper sauce, and simmer, loosely covered, until the chick-peas are tender, about 3 hours.

Puree the soup in a blender or food processor, reheat if necessary, and serve warm topped with the peanuts and cilantro or parsley for a lunch or dinner entrée soup.

MAKES 4 SERVINGS; 310 CALORIES PER SERVING; 10 GRAMS OF FAT; 29 PERCENT OF CALORIES FROM FAT.

lentil–sweet potato stew

Lentils are a good source of nerve-soothing B vitamins, as well as of magnesium and folate, making this a good dinner choice to help counteract a stressful autumn day.

1 tablespoon olive oil

3 cloves garlic, minced

1 onion, minced

3 teaspoons good-quality curry powder

1 teaspoon finely grated fresh gingerroot

1 fresh jalapeño pepper, seeded and minced

1 cup dried lentils

2 sweet potatoes, peeled and cubed

2 tomatoes, chopped, including juice

4 cups vegetable stock

Pinch of sea salt

1 cup plain nonfat yogurt or soy yogurt

¼ cup minced fresh cilantro or parsley

If the weather is damp: Use 2 jalapeños.

If the weather is dry: Chop 2 tomatoes and swirl them in along with the yogurt.

Heat a large soup pot on medium-high, and add the oil. Sauté the garlic, onion, curry powder, gingerroot, and jalapeño until the mixture is fragrant, about 4 minutes. Add the lentils, sweet potatoes, tomatoes, stock, and salt and bring to a boil. Reduce the heat to medium, cover loosely, and let the soup simmer until the lentils are tender, about 30 minutes. Swirl in the yogurt and sprinkle with the cilantro just before serving warm as an entrée soup.

MAKES 4 SERVINGS; 240 CALORIES PER SERVING; 4 GRAMS OF FAT; 15 PERCENT OF CALORIES FROM FAT.

red beans and barley

If the weather is damp:
Garnish each serving with
minced scallion.

————

If the weather is dry:
Garnish each serving with
chopped tomato.

The red kidney beans featured in this chili are a good source of digestion-toning fiber.

1 tablespoon olive oil

2 onions, chopped

3 cloves garlic, minced

1 jalapeño pepper, seeded and
    minced

1 tablespoon good-quality chili
    powder

Pinch of ground cinnamon

1 teaspoon dried oregano

2 cups chopped fresh tomatoes

1 cup vegetable stock

One 19-ounce can kidney beans,
    drained

1½ cups cooked barley

Heat a large soup pot on medium-high and add the oil. Sauté the onions, garlic, jalapeño, chili powder, cinnamon, and oregano until the onions have wilted and the mixture is fragrant, about 5 minutes.

Add the tomatoes, stock, beans, and barley and bring to a boil. Reduce the heat, cover loosely, and simmer until fragrant and slightly thickened, about 15 minutes. Serve warm as a lunch or dinner entrée.

MAKES 4 SERVINGS; 280 CALORIES PER SERVING; 5 GRAMS OF FAT; 15 PERCENT OF CALORIES FROM FAT.

black bean soup with epazote

Epazote, which is used in Mexican bean dishes to relieve intestinal gas, perfumes this thick and fragrant repast with a strong, thymelike aroma.

½ pound dried black turtle beans

1 quart vegetable stock

1 bay leaf

1 teaspoon good-quality
   chili powder, or to taste

1 teaspoon cuminseed

1 teaspoon coriander seed

1 tablespoon minced fresh oregano,
   or 1½ teaspoons dried

3 cloves garlic, peeled

1 tablespoon olive oil

1 onion, chopped

Juice of 1 lime

¼ cup minced celery leaf

2 tablespoons dried epazote
   (available at specialty food stores)

2 tablespoons Worcestershire sauce

Pinch of sea salt

If the weather is damp: Garnish the soup with minced scallion.

If the weather is dry: Garnish the soup with plain nonfat yogurt or soy yogurt.

Soak the beans in water to cover overnight. Discard the water.

In a large soup pot, combine the soaked beans, stock, and bay leaf and bring to a boil. Reduce the heat to a simmer, cover loosely, and simmer until the beans are just tender, about 1 hour.

Meanwhile, in a spice grinder or mortar, grind the chili powder, cuminseed, coriander seed, oregano, and garlic into a paste.

Heat a sauté pan on medium-high and add the olive oil. Add the paste, onion, lime juice, celery leaf, and epazote. Sauté until the mixture is fragrant, about 5 minutes.

When the beans are just about tender, scoop in the spice mixture along with the Worcestershire sauce and salt. Simmer gently for about 30 minutes more.

Let the beans cool, then transfer about 1½ cups to a food processor or blender and process until smooth. Stir the puree back into the soup and reheat. Serve warm as a lunch or dinner entrée.

MAKES 4 SERVINGS; 253 CALORIES PER SERVING; 6 GRAMS OF FAT; 21 PERCENT OF CALORIES FROM FAT.

rosemary-scented split pea soup

If the weather is damp: Garnish with minced fresh chives.

If the weather is dry: Serve with a lemon-dressed crisp green salad.

Like other legumes, split peas are a good source of healthy dietary fiber. But unlike other legumes, split peas contain only a trace of fat, making them a good choice for autumn dieters.

2 cups dried split peas
10 cups vegetable stock
2 cloves garlic, minced
1 onion, chopped
2 celery stalks, chopped, including leaves
4 carrots, chopped

1 large potato, chopped
1 bay leaf
1 tablespoon minced fresh rosemary, or 1½ teaspoons dried
Pinch of sea salt
Freshly ground black pepper to taste

In a large soup pot, combine the peas and stock and bring to a boil. Reduce the heat to a simmer and add the garlic, onion, celery, carrots, potato, bay leaf, and rosemary. Cover loosely and simmer until the peas are tender and the soup is thick, about 1½ hours, stirring occasionally. Stir in the salt and pepper and serve warm as a lunch or dinner entrée.

MAKES 4 SERVINGS; 296 CALORIES PER SERVING; LESS THAN 1 GRAM OF FAT; ABOUT 3 PERCENT OF CALORIES FROM FAT.

little bean cakes

I learned to make these in Zimbabwe, where they are eaten to fortify and nourish the body. Traditionally they are served as an accompaniment to roast meats, but I like them as a vegetarian entrée with roasted vegetables on the side.

If the weather is damp: Serve the cakes with a garnish of spicy salsa.

1½ cups cooked black-eyed peas
3 tablespoons minced fresh parsley
2 tablespoons minced red bell pepper
¼ cup minced onion
1 teaspoon minced fresh thyme, or ½ teaspoon dried
Freshly ground black pepper to taste
Pinch of sea salt

If the weather is dry: Serve the cakes with a garnish of plain nonfat yogurt or soy yogurt.

In a food processor or blender, puree the peas. Add the remaining ingredients and mix by hand until well combined.

Heat a large, well-seasoned dry cast-iron skillet on medium-high (use nonstick if you don't have cast iron). Form the pea mixture into 10 well-rounded, firm, tablespoon-sized balls. Flatten each between your hands and set 4 or 5 in the skillet. When brown, in about 2 minutes, flip them gently and brown on the other side. Repeat with the remaining cakes. Serve warm for lunch or dinner.

MAKES 10 LITTLE CAKES, OR ABOUT 4 SERVINGS; 180 CALORIES PER SERVING; LESS THAN 1 GRAM OF FAT; ABOUT 5 PERCENT OF CALORIES FROM FAT.

white bean spread with basil

If the weather is damp: Be liberal with the hot pepper sauce. Then spread on toasted whole wheat pita bread or whole wheat English muffins.

If the weather is dry: Add about ¼ cup vegetable stock when pureeing, and use as a dip for fresh vegetables.

The beans in this fiber-packed spread are a good source of folate, a nutrient that may help banish autumn depression.

1 cup cooked white beans
2 cloves garlic, minced
2 scallions, chopped
2 teaspoons olive oil
1 teaspoon minced fresh basil, or
   ½ teaspoon dried

½ teaspoon hot pepper sauce, or
   to taste
Pinch of sea salt

In a food processor or blender, combine all of the ingredients and process until smooth. Serve as a snack, or as a lunch or dinner condiment.

MAKES ABOUT 1 CUP, OR SIXTEEN 1–TABLESPOON SERVINGS; 15 CALORIES PER SERVING; TRACE OF FAT.

lentil salad with lemon and fennel

Lentils are a good source of energizing saturated fat-free protein. This may be why, in India and the Middle East, folklore claims that lentils can lift sluggishness and depression.

1 cup dried lentils

3 cups vegetable stock or water

1 bay leaf

1 onion, minced

2 cloves garlic, minced

1 yellow bell pepper, cored and minced

2 celery stalks, minced, including leaves

2 tablespoons olive oil

Juice of 1 lemon

2 tablespoons fennel seeds

Pinch of sea salt

If the weather is damp: Add hot pepper sauce to taste to the dressing.

If the weather is dry: Serve the salad on nests of crisp lettuce.

In a large soup pot, combine the lentils, stock or water, and bay leaf and bring to a boil. Reduce the heat, cover loosely, and simmer until the lentils are just tender but not mushy, 20 to 25 minutes. Discard the bay leaf and strain and discard any excess stock.

Transfer the lentils to a serving bowl and add the onion, garlic, bell pepper, and celery.

In a small bowl, whisk together the oil and the lemon juice. Heat a dry sauté pan on medium-high and add the fennel seeds, stirring until fragrant and toasted, about 2 minutes. Stir the seeds into the dressing along with the salt, and pour over the lentils, tossing well to combine. Serve warm or at room temperature as a lunch or dinner entrée.

MAKES 4 SERVINGS; 265 CALORIES PER SERVING; 7 GRAMS OF FAT; 24 PERCENT OF CALORIES FROM FAT.

wild rice with toasted pine nuts

If the weather is damp: Be liberal with the dry mustard.

If the weather is dry: Serve on a nest of crisp lettuce.

Wild rice is a good autumn food, providing the mineral zinc for immune function and upper respiratory health. This is a great dish to take to parties—it's tasty and festive.

1 cup uncooked wild rice

4 cups water

1 bay leaf

2 tablespoons pine nuts

1 red bell pepper, cored and thinly sliced

1 yellow bell pepper, cored and thinly sliced

2 scallions, minced

2 cloves garlic, minced

1 shallot, minced

2 tablespoons minced fresh basil, or 2 teaspoons dried

1 teaspoon minced fresh thyme, or 1 teaspoon dried

2 tablespoons balsamic vinegar

1 tablespoon lemon juice

2 teaspoons olive oil

Pinch of dry mustard

Pinch of sea salt

Freshly ground black pepper to taste

2 tablespoons crumbled feta cheese or crumbled blanched tofu (page 211)

In a large soup pot, combine the rice, water, and bay leaf and boil, uncovered, until the rice is tender but still a bit chewy, about 35 minutes. Drain the excess water and discard the bay leaf.

Meanwhile, heat a dry sauté pan on medium-high and add the pine nuts. Shake the pan over the heat for 2 to 3 minutes, until the nuts have toasted.

When the rice is ready, transfer it to a large bowl along with the pine nuts, bell peppers, scallions, garlic, shallot, basil, and thyme.

In a small bowl, whisk together the vinegar, lemon juice, oil, mustard, salt, and pepper. Pour it over the rice mixture and toss well to combine. Serve warm or at room temperature, sprinkled with the feta, for a lunch or dinner entrée.

MAKES 4 SERVINGS; 170 CALORIES PER SERVING; 6 GRAMS OF FAT; 33 PERCENT OF CALORIES FROM FAT.

rice with corn and lentils

Brown rice contains niacin, thiamine, and vitamin B_6, all essential to maintain energy levels, especially as the days grow shorter.

2 teaspoons olive oil

2 carrots, diced

1 red bell pepper, cored and diced

1 leek, topped, tailed, and thinly sliced

¾ cup uncooked brown rice

¼ cup dried lentils

2 cups vegetable stock or water

1 bay leaf

Pinch of sea salt

1 tablespoon minced fresh oregano, or 1½ teaspoons dried

1 cup fresh corn kernels

If the weather is damp: Add cayenne to taste when stirring in the corn, and serve warm.

If the weather is dry: Serve at room temperature topped with chopped fresh tomatoes.

Heat a large soup pot on medium-high. Add the oil and sauté the carrots, bell pepper, and leek until they're fragrant and just wilted, about 2 minutes. Add the rice and lentils, continuing to sauté for another 2 minutes. Add the stock or water and bay leaf and bring to a boil. Reduce the heat to medium-low, cover loosely, and simmer gently until the rice is tender, about 30 minutes. Stir in the salt, oregano, and corn; heat through, and serve warm or at room temperature as a lunch or dinner entrée.

MAKES 4 SERVINGS; 260 CALORIES PER SERVING; 4 GRAMS OF FAT; 14 PERCENT OF CALORIES FROM FAT.

barley "risotto" with leeks

If the weather is damp: Increase the garlic to 3 cloves.

Leek contains the same healthful sulfur compounds as its cousins garlic and onion. It is popular in Wales and in northern England, where residents have been heard to say, "If you can't get an onion, take a leek."

If the weather is dry: Add a stalk of minced celery, including leaves, when you add the carrots.

1 cup uncooked barley
2 teaspoons olive oil
2 carrots, minced
2 leeks, topped, tailed, and minced
2 cloves garlic, minced
1 bay leaf

1 teaspoon minced fresh rosemary, or ½ teaspoon dried
Pinch of sea salt
3 cups vegetable stock

Heat a large soup pot on medium-high and add the barley, stirring constantly until fragrant and lightly browned, about 4 minutes. Add the oil, carrots, leeks, garlic, bay leaf, and rosemary and continue to sauté until the vegetables are slightly wilted, about 3 minutes. Add the salt and stock and bring to a boil.

Reduce the heat, cover loosely, and simmer until the barley is tender, about 35 minutes. Serve warm as a lunch or dinner entrée.

MAKES 4 SERVINGS; 205 CALORIES PER SERVING; 3 GRAMS OF FAT; 13 PERCENT OF CALORIES FROM FAT.

carrot coins with garlic, lemon, and basil

This would be an apt dish for those suffering from a cold, since the beta carotene in the carrots can help deter mucus production.

1 pound carrots, cut into coins

2 teaspoons olive oil

2 cloves garlic, minced

2 tablespoons minced fresh basil, or
  1 teaspoon dried

1 tablespoon lemon juice

Pinch of sea salt

Freshly ground black pepper to taste

If the weather is damp: Be liberal with the black pepper.

If the weather is dry: Double the lemon juice.

Pour an inch of water into a saucepan and bring to a boil. Add the carrots, cover loosely, and simmer until just tender, about 4 minutes. Drain the carrots and pat them dry.

Heat a sauté pan on medium-high. Add the oil and sauté the carrots, garlic, basil, lemon juice, salt, and pepper until the mixture is fragrant and heated through, about 2 minutes. Serve warm or at room temperature as a side dish.

MAKES 4 SERVINGS; 70 CALORIES PER SERVING; 2.5 GRAMS OF FAT; 32 PERCENT OF CALORIES FROM FAT.

thyme-roasted vegetables

If the weather is damp: Sprinkle with freshly ground black pepper before serving.

If the weather is dry: Add 2 chopped tomatoes, including juice, to the vegetable mixture before roasting.

Thyme contains a compound called thymol that can help clear a stuffy head, making this a perfect dish for those with congestion.

4 carrots, sliced

2 onions, quartered

2 cups whole button mushrooms

2 medium potatoes, cut into 2-inch chunks

5 cloves garlic, peeled

2 teaspoons olive oil

1 bay leaf

1 tablespoon minced fresh thyme, or 1 teaspoon dried

Pinch of sea salt

1½ cups vegetable stock or water

Preheat the oven to 400°F.

In a large cast-iron roaster, or other roasting pan, combine all of the ingredients and cover. Roast until the vegetables are almost tender, about 45 minutes. Remove the cover, stir, and continue to roast, uncovered, until the vegetables are very tender, about 20 minutes more. Serve warm as a lunch or dinner entrée.

MAKES 4 SERVINGS; 192 CALORIES PER SERVING; 2.25 GRAMS OF FAT; 12 PERCENT OF CALORIES FROM FAT.

savory corn and onion pudding

Chili powder, which perfumes this piquant dish, contains volatile oils that help increase circulation and thus warm the body.

4 egg whites, or 2 whole eggs, or
  ½ cup commercial egg substitute,
  beaten
1½ cups skim milk, whole milk, or
  plain nonfat soy milk
1 teaspoon good-quality chili
  powder

Pinch of sea salt
Splash of hot pepper sauce, or
  to taste
1 cup fresh corn kernels
2 onions, chopped

If the weather is damp: Add a minced jalapeño to the mixture before baking.

If the weather is dry: Serve with fresh orange or tangerine sections.

Preheat the oven to 350°F. Lightly oil a soufflé dish.

In a large bowl, whisk together the eggs and milk. Stir in the remaining ingredients.

Pour the mixture into the prepared soufflé dish and bake until the pudding is firm and lightly browned on top, about 1 hour. Serve warm for breakfast, brunch, or lunch.

MAKES 4 SERVINGS; 80 CALORIES PER SERVING (WITH EGG WHITES AND SKIM MILK); TRACE OF FAT.

grilled onion brochettes

If the weather is damp:
Add a splash of hot pepper
sauce to the marinade.

———

If the weather is dry:
Remove the onions from
the skewers and toss with
chopped tomato. Serve
room temperature as a
salad on a bed of curly red
lettuce.

This is a warming choice for a chilly autumn eve. As a bonus, the lemon and rosemary make the onions more digestible.

1 pound tiny onions in their skins (about 16)
Juice of 1 lemon
Pinch of sea salt

Pinch of cayenne
1 teaspoon minced fresh rosemary, or ½ teaspoon dried

Blanch the onions in boiling water until they're barely tender, about 5 minutes. Then drain and pat dry.

When the onions are cool enough to handle, peel them, leaving the root end on so they won't fall apart on the skewer.

In a large bowl, combine the onions, lemon juice, salt, pepper, and rosemary and marinate for at least an hour, but overnight is best.

When you're ready, preheat the grill or broiler. Thread the onions on bamboo skewers and grill or broil until the brochettes are fragrant and mahogany in color, about 5 minutes, turning the skewers so the onions are cooked on all sides. Serve warm as a side dish for lunch or dinner. Leftovers are delicious tossed with balsamic vinegar and served slightly chilled on a nest of crisp greens.

MAKES 4 SERVINGS; 33 CALORIES PER SERVING; NO ADDED FAT.

baked onions with pumpkin

Pumpkin is an abundant source of beta carotene, the plant form of resistance-building vitamin A.

One 2½-pound jack-o'-lantern–type pumpkin

2 onions, chopped

1 baking apple, such as Granny Smith, peeled, cored, and chopped

Pinch of ground cinnamon

Pinch of sea salt

If the weather is damp: Increase the amount of ground cinnamon.

If the weather is dry: Stir in 1 tablespoon lemon juice before baking.

Preheat the oven to 375°F.

Cut the top off the pumpkin and use a large spoon to scrape out and discard the seeds. Fill the pumpkin with the onions, apple, cinnamon, and salt and stir to mix. Cover with the top of the pumpkin. If the top has a stem, cover it with foil so it won't burn. Set the pumpkin in a baking dish, such as a 9-inch cake pan, and bake until the pumpkin is tender, about 2 hours. Open the pumpkin and serve warm as a side dish, making sure to scoop out some pumpkin along with the onions.

MAKES 4 SERVINGS; 40 CALORIES PER SERVING; NO ADDED FAT.

stuffed vidalia onions

*If the weather is damp:
Add a clove of minced
garlic to the puree.*

*If the weather is dry: Add
½ teaspoon lemon zest to
the puree.*

The onions are filled with pureed collards, which are a good source of nerve-soothing calcium.

4 large Vidalia or Spanish onions
½ cup vegetable stock
One 10-ounce package collard
   greens, thawed and well drained
1 tablespoon minced fresh oregano,
   or 1 teaspoon dried

¼ cup crumbled feta cheese or
   blanched tofu (page 211)
2 tablespoons bread crumbs
Olive oil for rubbing

Preheat the oven to 450°F. Lightly oil a baking dish.

Peel the onions and chop off a slice at the bottom so they can sit without rolling. Then use a melon baller to scoop out the insides of each onion, taking about ½ cup from each one. Chop the scooped-out parts and add them, with the stock, to a large skillet. Simmer until the onions have wilted, about 5 minutes. Scoop the mixture into a food processor or blender and puree. While the motor is running add the collards, oregano, cheese, and bread crumbs. When the mixture is smooth, use a teaspoon to pack it into the onion globes. If you have leftover puree, scoop it into a small, lightly oiled baking dish and bake it when you bake the onions.

Rub the outside of each onion with a bit of olive oil and set into the prepared baking dish. Bake until the onions are tender, 20 to 25 minutes. Serve warm as a lunch or dinner side dish.

MAKES 4 SERVINGS; 55 CALORIES PER SERVING; 2 GRAMS OF FAT; 33 PERCENT OF CALORIES FROM FAT.

sesame sticks

This crunchy snack is an easy way to incorporate the protective properties of garlic and onion into your autumn diet. It is great for after-school snacks or for a tasty office repast.

¾ cup whole wheat pastry flour

½ cup unbleached flour

¼ cup grated Parmesan cheese or soy Parmesan

1 teaspoon finely grated onion

2 cloves garlic, very finely minced

Pinch of cayenne, or to taste

1 tablespoon sesame seeds

¼ cup olive oil

About ¼ cup ice water

If the weather is damp: Use 3 garlic cloves instead of 2.

If the weather is dry: Enjoy with a glass of orange juice.

Preheat the oven to 375°F. Lightly oil an open-sided cookie sheet.

In a medium bowl, combine the flours, cheese, onion, garlic, cayenne, and seeds. Form a well in the center and pour in the oil, stirring to blend. Add the cold water gradually, tablespoon by tablespoon, mixing with your hands until you can form the dough into a ball.

Place the dough on the prepared cookie sheet and roll into a 15 × 10-inch rectangle. With a pastry wheel or pizza cutter, cut the dough into 1 × 1½-inch strips.

Bake the sticks until they're crisp and golden, 18 to 20 minutes. Carefully remove the sticks from the cookie sheet and let them cool on a wire rack. Store in a tightly closed tin or plastic container for up to 1 week. Enjoy as a snack.

MAKES 6 SERVINGS; 180 CALORIES PER SERVING; 11 GRAMS OF FAT; 50 PERCENT OF CALORIES FROM FAT.

greens
leafy elixirs

At the Thursday market in Harare, Zimbabwe, a woman showed me two ways in which she prepared autumn greens. Collards, kale, turnip greens, and beet greens can all be rinsed, cut into strips, and simmered in lightly salted water until they are bright green and tender, she said. It should take only four to five minutes, or slightly longer if the greens are large and tough. The Zimbabwe woman tossed the drained, still-warm greens with chopped tomato and garlic before eating, and indeed it is a delicious combination.

The second technique was to dry the greens, for which she arranged the fresh strips in a single layer on a large, oval, wooden tray. The tray was placed in a shady spot, where it took the greens about three days to dry. She stored the shriveled strips in covered glass jars, adding them to soups and stews when fresh greens were unavailable.

Greens are an important supplier of immune-enhancing vitamins and minerals in the Zimbabwe diet, and some people eat them, fresh or dried, every day. Research in science and medicine in the West supports that greens are an important disease-fighting tonic, containing carotene compounds to fight colds and flu, calcium to strengthen the nervous system, and chlorophyll to tone the digestive system. Half a pound of fresh greens makes one serving of cooked greens, or about half a cup, containing about 25 calories and virtually no fat.

While munching your collards and kale, ponder that in the folklore of many cultures the color green is a symbol of abundance, longevity, health, and wisdom. Since much that sprouts from the earth is green, the color often stands for freedom and the breaking of shackles.

quick cooking tip for greens

For greens in a flash, rinse, slice, and loosely pack about two cups of (still wet) greens in a two-cup measure. Cover with vented plastic wrap and microwave on full power until they're bright green and just wilted, two to three minutes, depending on the toughness of the greens. Use in your favorite greens recipe, or drain, pat dry, and toss with sesame oil and soy sauce for a tasty side dish.

garlic-steamed greens

If the weather is damp:
Add hot pepper sauce to
taste when you add the
lemon juice.

———

If the weather is dry:
Increase the lemon juice to
3 tablespoons.

The beta carotene from the greens, combined with the sulfur compounds in the garlic and scallions, makes this the perfect autumn dish for temporarily clearing sinuses.

1 pound fresh collards or kale, cut
    into strips
3 cloves garlic, thinly sliced
2 scallions, minced

2 tablespoons fresh lemon juice
Pinch of sea salt
Freshly ground black pepper to taste

Combine the greens and garlic in a steamer basket, cover, and steam over boiling water until they're tender, 4 to 5 minutes. In a medium bowl, combine the greens and garlic with the scallions, lemon juice, salt, and pepper, and serve warm as a side dish for lunch or dinner.

MAKES 2 LARGE SERVINGS; 30 CALORIES PER SERVING; NO ADDED FAT.

warm greens with sesame dressing

The gingerroot in the dressing adds a snap to the "bite" of the greens. In addition, gingerroot contains volatile oils that help to stimulate digestion and warm the body.

If the weather is damp: Double the amount of gingerroot.

1 pound fresh collards or kale, cut into strips
1 teaspoon tahini (sesame butter)
1 teaspoon miso (available at natural food stores and Asian markets)

2 tablespoons lemon juice
1 teaspoon finely minced fresh gingerroot

If the weather is dry: Toss with 2 cups just-cooked pasta and serve warm.

Steam the greens over boiling water until they're tender, 4 to 5 minutes.

Meanwhile, in a medium bowl, whisk together the remaining ingredients. When the greens are ready, add them to the bowl and toss well to combine. Serve warm as a lunch or dinner side dish.

MAKES 2 SERVINGS; 54 CALORIES PER SERVING; TRACE OF FAT.

zesty greens

If the weather is damp: Serve the greens as open-faced sandwiches on crusty whole-grain bread.

If the weather is dry: Swirl the greens into 2 cups warm rice.

Think of this as a "cooked" salad. It has similar ingredients and nutrients, but the steaming and sautéing warms it for autumn.

2 pounds collards or kale, chopped

1 teaspoon olive oil

1 large onion, chopped

2 cloves garlic, minced

½ pound plum tomatoes, peeled and chopped (drain if using canned)

¼ cup minced fresh parsley

1 tablespoon balsamic vinegar

1 teaspoon hot pepper sauce, or to taste

Pinch of sea salt

Steam the greens over boiling water until they're tender, 4 to 5 minutes. Drain well and pat dry.

Heat a medium sauté pan on medium-high heat and add the oil. Sauté the onion and garlic until they're fragrant and soft, about 7 minutes. Add the tomatoes, parsley, vinegar, hot pepper sauce, and salt and simmer for about 4 minutes. Add the greens and heat through for about 1 minute. Serve as a side dish for lunch or dinner.

MAKES 4 SERVINGS; 66 CALORIES PER SERVING; 1 GRAM OF FAT; 14 PERCENT OF CALORIES FROM FAT.

green elixir

This tonic makes a great soup stock. But I also like to sip it warm in a heavy mug as an autumn restorative. It's great to serve to weary friends and travelers.

1 pound collards, kale, or other fall greens, chopped

3 cloves garlic, peeled
Pinch of sea salt

Set the greens in a large soup pot and pour on water to cover. Add the garlic and salt and bring to a boil. Reduce the heat to low, cover loosely, and let the greens simmer for 1½ hours. Discard the greens and garlic and sip the reviving brew warm, or use it as a soup stock or base for sauces.

MAKES 1¼ QUARTS, ABOUT TEN ½-CUP SERVINGS; ABOUT 5 CALORIES PER SERVING; NO ADDED FAT.

If the weather is damp: Add a splash of hot pepper sauce before drinking.

If the weather is dry: Add a splash of lemon juice before drinking.

soup with greens and orzo

Light and easy to digest, this soup will leave you nicely energized for autumn evening activities.

1 quart vegetable stock
½ cup orzo or other tiny pasta
1 cup very finely chopped fresh kale or collards

2 cloves garlic, peeled
Pinch of sea salt

In a large soup pot, bring the stock to a boil. Add the rest of the ingredients and continue to boil until the orzo is tender and the greens are bright in color, about 5 minutes. Serve warm any time of day.

MAKES 4 SERVINGS; 75 CALORIES PER SERVING; NO ADDED FAT.

If the weather is damp: Sprinkle with freshly ground black pepper and serve the soup in warmed bowls.

If the weather is dry: Add 2 chopped tomatoes to the soup before serving.

green sauce
(for tofu, tempeh, pasta, rice, barley, or fish)

If the weather is damp: Swirl ¼ cup of the sauce into a cup of spicy vegetable soup before serving.

If the weather is dry: Pour ½ cup of the sauce in a pool on a plate and set a piece of poached tofu or salmon atop.

Seasonal greens and fragrant herbs combine to illuminate your autumn entrées.

1 pound collards or kale, chopped
  and steamed
¼ cup fresh parsley
¼ cup fresh basil

1 tablespoon minced fresh chives
Pinch of sea salt
½ cup vegetable stock or water

In a food processor or blender, combine all of the ingredients and puree.

MAKES ENOUGH FOR 4 SERVINGS; 25 CALORIES PER SERVING; NO ADDED FAT.

orange-fleshed squash
sweet sustenance

At an October Hopi powwow in Arizona, I was served plain baked squash after a meal, instead of a gooey dessert. Perhaps this tradition began because of the absence of sugar in the desert. But Hopi cooks continue to serve baked squash at meal's end to honor the vegetable. Squash is a Hopi symbol to inspire crops, and by serving it at the end of a meal, the flow of food is symbolically encouraged. Hopi cooks use dried, hollow squashes as water vessels, and filled with pebbles as rattles to encourage rain. Along with beans and corn, squash is one of the "three sisters," daughters of the Earth Mother and the foundation of Hopi cooking.

Squash is a nutritious as well as a symbolic foundation, since its flesh is an excellent source of immune-enhancing beta carotene. Half a cup, cooked, contains between 40 and 60 calories, depending on the variety, and provides digestion-friendly fiber and energizing carbohydrates.

select a squash

Hubbard, Butternut, Acorn, Boston, Turban, Delicata, and Buttercup are all varieties of orange-fleshed squash. Sometimes called "winter" squash because they come to hard-shelled maturity on the vine in cool weather, these tasty squash originally come from South America.

quick cooking tip for squash

Chop a pound of peeled, orange-fleshed squash into one-inch pieces and arrange in a one-quart baking dish with two tablespoons of orange juice and a bay leaf. Cover with vented plastic wrap and microwave on full power until the squash is tender, about four minutes. Drain and use in your favorite squash recipe, or puree to use instead of pumpkin in a pie.

squash with millet

If the weather is damp: Add 1 teaspoon finely grated fresh gingerroot before cooking.

If the weather is dry: Garnish with minced fresh scallions.

Squash and millet are sweet-tasting and thus can help neutralize a sour autumn stomach. Iroquois folklore holds that squash can neutralize a sour disposition, as well.

1 cup yellow millet
1 cup squash, peeled and cut into
   1-inch chunks (about ½ pound)

3 cups vegetable stock or water
Pinch of sea salt

In a medium saucepan, combine all of the ingredients and bring to a boil. Reduce the heat to medium-low, cover loosely, and simmer until the millet is tender, stirring occasionally, about 35 minutes. Serve warm as porridge for breakfast or brunch, or as a lunch or dinner side dish.

MAKES 4 LARGE SERVINGS; 127 CALORIES PER SERVING; NO ADDED FAT.

spiced squash puree

Cardamom, allspice, and coriander, which perfume this dish, are what herbalists call "aromatics," substances that gently soothe digestion.

1 large butternut squash, peeled, seeded, and chunked (or 1½ pounds of any orange-fleshed squash you like)
1 teaspoon ground coriander seeds

3 allspice berries, ground
Seeds of 2 cardamom pods, ground
1 tablespoon pure maple syrup
2 teaspoons unsalted butter
Pinch of sea salt

If the weather is damp: Add 1 teaspoon finely grated fresh gingerroot while pureeing.

If the weather is dry: Add 2 teaspoons fresh lime juice while pureeing.

Steam the squash over boiling water until it's very tender, 15 to 20 minutes. Tip into a food processor or blender along with the remaining ingredients and puree. Serve warm as an accompaniment to grilled tofu or fish.

MAKES 4 SERVINGS; 70 CALORIES PER SERVING; 2.1 GRAMS OF FAT; 27 PERCENT OF CALORIES FROM FAT.

squash with almonds and thyme

Thyme contains thymol, which has antiseptic and antibacterial properties that can help deter autumn colds and flu.

1 butternut squash, peeled, seeded, and cubed (or 1½ pounds of any orange-fleshed squash you like)
2 tablespoons sliced almonds

2 teaspoons minced fresh thyme, or 1 teaspoon dried
Pinch of sea salt

If the weather is damp: Add freshly ground pepper before serving.

If the weather is dry: Add 1 tablespoon fresh lemon juice to the sauté pan.

Steam the squash over boiling water until it's just tender, about 10 minutes. In a large dry sauté pan, combine the almonds, thyme, salt, and steamed squash and heat on high until the mixture is fragrant and the squash has dried off from steaming, 2 to 3 minutes. Serve warm as a lunch or dinner side dish.

MAKES 4 SERVINGS; 70 CALORIES PER SERVING; 1.75 GRAMS OF FAT; 22 PERCENT OF CALORIES FROM FAT.

hot peppers
pungent potion

As a morning beverage at a spa in California, I was offered a mug of hot water, lemon juice, and cayenne. The "hot stuff," the staff herbalist explained, contains a crystalline substance called "capsaicin," a compound that activates digestion by stimulating saliva and the flow of gastric juices. In addition, hot peppers or chile peppers, such as cayenne and its several hundred relations, provide a feeling of internal warmth and mild stimulation—good qualities to balance a cool autumn.

For centuries, African, Mexican, Indonesian, and East Indian herbalists have recommended hot peppers as digestive tonics to fight flatulence, constipation, and dyspepsia. Hot peppers are eaten in cool weather to provide internal heat, or Uncle Ho's coveted "yang belly."

the measure of heat

The "hot" in hot peppers is measured in Scoville units. For instance, habanero is a very hot variety of pepper, measuring 250,000 units. Jalapeño is a much milder variety, measuring 5,500 units.

quick cooking tips for hot peppers

Use dried, ground hot pepper by adding a pinch to a cup of citrus tea or to a cup of vegetable soup. Stir a teaspoon of hot pepper flakes into a pot of soup or stew to serve four. Or add one minced fresh hot pepper to a stir-fry to serve four, noting that the seeds and ribs contain maximum heat, and should be added or withheld according to your taste.

For a smoky, mellow flavor, roast fresh hot peppers as you would bell peppers: sear them under the broiler or on a grill, rotating frequently, until the skins are charred. Place the peppers in a large bowl and cover with a tea towel until cool. Using gloves, remove and discard the skins, cores, and tops.

hot sauce

The thermogenic (heat) nature of this spicy tonic helps to increase metabolism and circulation while warming the body.

25 fresh hot peppers, seeded and chopped (use gloves)
3 onions, sliced
5 cloves garlic, minced

6 cups chopped tomatoes (about 12 tomatoes)
3 cups cider vinegar
½ cup honey

If the weather is damp: This sauce is perfect.

If the weather is dry: Serve with moist foods such as pasta or barley.

In a large pot, combine the hot peppers, onions, garlic, tomatoes, and vinegar and bring to a boil. Continue to boil until the vegetables are tender, about 15 minutes. Discard the vegetables, stir in the honey, and boil until the sauce has thickened, about 15 minutes more.

To store, let the sauce cool, then refrigerate for up to a month. To use, swirl ¼ cup (or to taste) into a chili, soup, stew, casserole, sauté, or stir-fry to serve 4. Or use as a table condiment, drizzled to taste on rice, beans, steamed vegetables, tofu, or fish.

MAKES ABOUT 3½ CUPS, OR FOURTEEN ¼-CUP SERVINGS; 77 CALORIES PER SERVING; NO ADDED FAT.

hot pepper salsa

If the weather is damp:
Use the larger amount of
hot peppers and garlic.

If the weather is dry:
Substitute I tablespoon
fresh lime juice for the
vinegar.

Try this tasty potion as an autumn midafternoon reviver.

1 tablespoon minced fresh cilantro
2 bell peppers, roasted (page 287) and chopped
1 to 2 cloves garlic, minced
1 to 2 fresh hot peppers, seeded (use gloves)

½ teaspoon ground cuminseed
1 teaspoon minced fresh oregano
½ teaspoon honey
1 tablespoon balsamic vinegar
Pinch of sea salt

In a food processor or blender, combine all of the ingredients and process until combined but still slightly chunky. Serve with baked corn chips or corn bread, or atop a poached egg.

MAKES ABOUT ½ CUP, OR TWO ¼-CUP SERVINGS; 66 CALORIES PER SERVING; NO ADDED FAT.

roasted peppers with chile and basil

If the weather is damp:
Sprinkle with freshly
ground pepper before
enjoying.

If the weather is dry:
Substitute fresh lemon
juice for the vinegar.

Peppers, sweet bell and hot, are a good source of immune-boosting vitamin C.

4 large bell peppers, roasted (page 287) and sliced
2 tablespoons minced fresh basil
2 teaspoons balsamic vinegar

1 fresh hot pepper, seeded and minced (use gloves)
Pinch of sea salt

In a medium bowl, combine all of the ingredients and toss well to combine. Serve at room temperature as a salad or as an open-faced sandwich on crusty bread.

MAKES 4 SERVINGS; 40 CALORIES PER SERVING; NO ADDED FAT.

spicy bean burritos

The pungent nature of this dish makes it a mildly energizing autumn lunch. What's more, it packs well for traveling to office, school, or picnics.

1 tablespoon olive oil

1 onion, minced

1 clove garlic, minced

4 bell peppers, roasted (page 287) and chopped

1½ cups cooked or canned pinto beans

2 fresh hot peppers, seeded and minced (use gloves)

1 tablespoon minced fresh oregano, or 1½ teaspoons dried

4 wheat tortillas

½ cup nonfat ricotta or soft soy cheese

If the weather is damp: Serve topped with Hot Pepper Salsa (page 288).

If the weather is dry: Serve with fresh chopped tomatoes and lettuce.

Heat a large sauté pan on medium-high, and add the oil. Sauté the onion and garlic until they're fragrant and soft, about 5 minutes. Add the roasted peppers, beans, hot peppers, and oregano and sauté for about 2 minutes more.

Place a tortilla in a dry cast-iron or other heavy skillet and heat on medium, turning frequently until the tortilla is soft and pliable. Repeat with the remaining 3 tortillas. Spread about ¼ cup of filling down the center of a tortilla in a band 4 inches long and 1 inch wide. Over it spread about 1 tablespoon of cheese. Turn one end in, fold one long side over the filling, and roll up. Set the burrito in a baking dish in a warm oven while you repeat the filling with the remaining tortillas. Serve warm as a lunch or dinner entrée.

MAKES 4 BURRITOS; 175 CALORIES EACH; 4 GRAMS OF FAT; 21 PERCENT OF CALORIES FROM FAT.

warming sauce
(for pasta, fish, tempeh, seitan, or tofu)

If the weather is damp: Be generous with the hot pepper sauce.

If the weather is dry: Substitute fresh lemon juice for the vinegar.

The gentle heat properties of garlic, hot peppers, and rosemary are a good way to end a chilly autumn day.

5 red bell peppers, roasted
  (page 287) and minced
2 teaspoons olive oil
2 cloves garlic, minced
1 teaspoon capers, mashed
1 teaspoon minced fresh rosemary,
  or ½ teaspoon dried and crushed

1 teaspoon hot pepper sauce, or
  to taste
1 tablespoon balsamic vinegar
Pinch of sea salt

In a medium bowl, combine all of the ingredients, cover, and let the sauce meld at room temperature for 1 hour. Toss with enough hot pasta or rice to serve 4 (about 4 cups, cooked), or heat the sauce gently before drizzling over grilled fish or tofu.

MAKES 4 SERVINGS OF SAUCE; 75 CALORIES PER SERVING; 2 GRAMS OF FAT; 24 PERCENT OF CALORIES FROM FAT.

chile-steamed vegetables

Fresh jalapeño pepper adds warmth and digestibility to nutritious autumn greens.

1 pound fresh kale or collards, sliced into strips
3 cloves garlic, thinly sliced

1 fresh jalapeño, seeded and minced
1 tablespoon fresh lemon juice
Pinch of sea salt

If the weather is damp: Use 2 jalapeños.

If the weather is dry: Increase the lemon juice to 2 tablespoons. Or, use ½ pound greens and ½ pound very thinly sliced potatoes.

Steam the greens, garlic, and jalapeño, covered, over boiling water until the greens are tender and bright green, 6 to 8 minutes. If the greens are very water-logged, press out the water between 2 plates, taking care not to lose the garlic and jalapeño. Toss with the lemon juice and sea salt and serve warm as a side dish or tucked into a toasted whole wheat pita.

MAKES 2 LARGE SERVINGS; 30 CALORIES PER SERVING; NO ADDED FAT.

chili-topped potatoes

If the weather is damp: Add hot pepper sauce to taste to the vegetables while sautéing.

If the weather is dry: Use 2 tomatoes.

Chili powder, oregano, and fresh hot peppers lighten the sometimes heavy digestibility of filled baked potatoes.

1 bell pepper, seeded and chopped
⅓ cup fresh corn kernels
1 onion, chopped
1 tomato, chopped
1 or 2 fresh jalapeños, seeded and minced
1 or 2 cloves garlic, minced

1 teaspoon chili powder, or to taste
2 teaspoons minced fresh oregano, or 1 teaspoon dried
Pinch of sea salt
¼ cup vegetable stock or water
4 potatoes, baked

In a large sauté pan, combine all the ingredients except the potatoes and sauté on medium-high until the stock has boiled away and the vegetables are fragrant and just tender, about 3 minutes.

Split open the potatoes and scoop an equal amount of the vegetable mixture onto each. Serve warm as a lunch or dinner entrée.

MAKES 4 SERVINGS; 260 CALORIES PER SERVING; NO ADDED FAT.

apples and pears
fall fruits for fitness

A Norwegian herbalist told me that health-minded people in her country follow the "apple diet" each autumn. For one whole day they eat nothing but apples—fresh, dried, sauced, or juiced, the object being to "clean" the intestines, preparing them for a healthy fall season. And if perchance they run out of apples, pears can substitute.

The logic in the "apple diet" may come from the fact that apples and pears are excellent sources of insoluble fiber, which promotes digestive health, soothes diarrhea, corrects constipation, and helps prevent colon cancer. In addition, the fruits contain boron, a mineral that raises alertness levels, helping to reverse the tendency to become sluggish as the daylight hours diminish for the year.

apple allergy?

For some people, usually those who are allergic to aspirin, eating an apple causes itchy lips and mouths. If that's the case for you, peeling an apple before eating it raw, or opting for cooked apples, may be a solution.

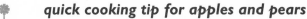

❋ quick cooking tip for apples and pears

For a fast and delicious autumn dessert, peel, core, and slice four apples or pears and arrange them in a large sauté pan with half a cup of apple juice, half a teaspoon of pumpkin pie spice, and a pinch of sea salt. Bring the mixture to a boil and simmer, stirring frequently, until the fruit is saucy and tender, about five minutes. Serve warm or chilled atop nonfat vanilla yogurt, or a lemony cake.

cinnamon-poached fruit

If the weather is damp: Add a whole cinnamon stick to the tea during simmering.

If the weather is dry: Add half a sliced fresh orange to the tea during simmering.

Cinnamon's warm, sharp nature is a mild digestive tonic, helping those who bloat from eating apples and pears to enjoy them more comfortably.

3 apples, peeled, cored, and sliced

3 pears, peeled, cored, and sliced

2 cups brewed cinnamon tea

1 bay leaf

Pinch of sea salt

In a large frying pan, combine all of the ingredients and bring to a boil. Reduce the heat and simmer, uncovered, until the tea has been reduced by half and the fruit is tender, about 10 minutes. Serve warm or at room temperature for breakfast over hot cereal; or for dessert topped with nonfat vanilla yogurt (cow or soy). The fruit will keep, covered and refrigerated, for about 5 days; make it ahead and it will be ready for breakfast.

MAKES 4 SERVINGS; 137 CALORIES PER SERVING; NO ADDED FAT.

autumn fruits with creamy orange dressing

This simple salad is a good source of vitamin C and folate, to help build immunity against autumn respiratory infections.

2 apples, cored and sliced
1 pear, cored and sliced
2 pink grapefruit, peeled, sectioned, and seeded
1 cup plain nonfat yogurt or soy yogurt

2 tablespoons orange juice concentrate
Pinch of ground cinnamon

If the weather is damp: Be generous with the cinnamon.

If the weather is dry: Omit the cinnamon.

In a medium bowl, combine the apples, pear, and grapefruit. In a small bowl, gently mix together the yogurt, juice concentrate, and cinnamon. Scoop the yogurt over the fruit and toss well to combine.

MAKES 4 BREAKFAST, BRUNCH, SNACK, OR DESSERT SERVINGS; 130 CALORIES PER SERVING; NO ADDED FAT.

vanilla-poached pears

Scientists who study fragrance psychology say that vanilla's aroma is soothing and warming—fine qualities to balance a damp and chilly day.

2 large pears, peeled, halved, and cored
2 cups apple juice

1 cinnamon stick
1 vanilla bean, slit vertically

If the weather is damp: Serve the pears warm, in shallow bowls with their poaching juice, sprinkled with cinnamon.

If the weather is dry: Serve the pears very slightly chilled, in shallow bowls with their poaching juice, drizzled with lemon juice.

In a frying pan, combine all the ingredients and bring to a boil. Reduce the heat to a gentle simmer, cover loosely, and poach until tender, about 20 minutes. Let the pear halves relax in the juice for about 10 minutes before serving warm, or serve chilled in pretty dessert dishes.

MAKES 4 SERVINGS; 110 CALORIES PER SERVING; NO ADDED FAT.

apple-molasses bran muffins

If the weather is damp:
Add 1 teaspoon ground
cinnamon to the batter
before baking.

If the weather is dry:
Spread a muffin with apple
butter or pear butter
before enjoying.

These fat-free treats are a good source of digestion-friendly fiber.

1 cup wheat bran

1 cup buttermilk or nonfat soy milk, at room temperature

¾ cup whole wheat pastry flour

¾ cup unbleached flour

2 teaspoons baking powder

Pinch of sea salt

½ cup raisins

½ cup applesauce

3 egg whites, or ¼ cup plus 1 tablespoon commercial egg substitute, at room temperature

⅓ cup molasses

1 teaspoon pure vanilla extract

Preheat the oven to 375°F. Spray 2 muffin tins with nonstick spray.

Soak the bran in the milk for 10 minutes.

Meanwhile, in a large bowl, combine the flours, baking powder, sea salt, and raisins. In another bowl, combine the applesauce, egg whites or egg substitute, molasses, and vanilla extract. Add the soaked bran to the flour mixture, then stir in the molasses mixture and combine well. Don't overmix; about 15 strokes should do.

Scoop the batter into the prepared muffin tins. Bake until the muffins are cooked through, 18 to 22 minutes. Let the muffins cool in their tins for about 5 minutes, then transfer them to a wire rack to cool completely. Since they are made without added fat they will stay moist and delicious for only 1 day at room temperature, but you may freeze some and defrost as needed.

MAKES 12 MUFFINS; 115 CALORIES PER MUFFIN; NO ADDED FAT.

raisin-peanut squares

Here's an example of substituting digestion-friendly, fiber-rich apple butter for fat-laden butter in a cookie recipe.

1 cup raisins, minced

2 tablespoons natural peanut butter

1 pear, grated

¼ cup natural apple butter

⅓ cup pure maple syrup

2 egg whites, or ¼ cup commercial egg substitute, at room temperature

1 teaspoon pure vanilla extract

1 teaspoon grated orange peel

1 cup quick oats

¾ cup whole wheat pastry flour

¾ cup unbleached flour

Pinch of sea salt

If the weather is damp: Add ½ teaspoon ground cinnamon when you add the flours.

If the weather is dry: Serve with a cup of mint tea.

Preheat the oven to 375°F. Lightly oil an 8-inch square cake pan.

In a small bowl, combine the raisins and peanut butter and set aside. In a medium bowl, combine the remaining ingredients and mix well. The dough will be moist and slightly crumbly.

Press half the dough into the bottom of the cake pan with a floured hand, until the dough is smooth and without cracks. Firmly press the raisin mixture atop the dough. Then crumble the remaining half of the dough over the raisin layer, pressing it down firmly until it's smooth and without cracks.

Bake until the edges begin to turn brown, about 25 minutes. Let cool, then cut into 16 squares with a sharp knife.

MAKES 16 SQUARES; 163 CALORIES EACH; 1.5 GRAMS OF FAT; 8 PERCENT OF CALORIES FROM FAT.

chewy apple-oat bars

If the weather is damp:
Add ½ teaspoon ground
ginger when you add the
cinnamon.

If the weather is dry: Serve
with lemonade.

Oats are a good source of calming magnesium, as well as zinc for bolstering immunities to colds and flu.

1⅓ cups rolled oats	⅔ cup puffed rice cereal
⅓ cup raw sunflower seeds	½ cup pure maple syrup
½ teaspoon ground cinnamon	3 tablespoons pear butter
⅔ cup chopped dried apples	1 tablespoon unsalted butter

Preheat the oven to 325°F. Lightly oil an 8-inch square cake pan.

Put the oats and seeds into a dry 9 × 13-inch pan and toast in the oven, stirring frequently, for about 20 minutes. Remove them from the oven and pour them into a large bowl. Stir in the cinnamon, the dried apples, and the puffed rice.

In a small saucepan, combine the maple syrup, pear butter, and butter and bring to a boil, stirring frequently. Reduce the heat and simmer for 5 minutes, until the syrup has thickened. To test for doneness, dip the handle of a spoon into the hot mixture, which should feel warm but not sticky. Pour the syrup over the dry ingredients, stirring quickly, until they are well coated. Transfer to the square cake pan and press down firmly. Bake until firm, 20 to 25 minutes. Cool completely, then cut into 1 × 2-inch bars with a sharp knife. Store in a covered container for up to a week.

MAKES 24 BARS; 60 CALORIES PER BAR; 2 GRAMS OF FAT; 30 PERCENT OF CALORIES FROM FAT.

warm pear sauce

The silky texture of this sauce is soothing to a scratchy, sore throat.

4 ripe pears, peeled, cored, and chopped

6 dried apricots

½ cup orange juice

In a small saucepan, combine all of the ingredients and bring to a boil. Reduce the heat to medium-low and simmer until the fruit is fragrant and soft, about 4 minutes. Let cool for about 5 minutes, then scoop into a food processor or blender and puree. Serve atop pancakes, hot cereal, fruit salad, nonfat vanilla yogurt, or by itself.

MAKES ABOUT 1¼ CUPS, OR 2 LARGE SERVINGS; 220 CALORIES PER SERVING; NO ADDED FAT.

If the weather is damp: Add a pinch of freshly grated nutmeg to the ingredients before boiling.

If the weather is dry: Add 1 tablespoon lime juice to the ingredients before boiling; or stir in ¼ teaspoon pure vanilla extract after cooling.

STRENGTHENING AUTUMN MENUS

This season's best meals are comprised of slow-roasted or long-simmered recipes that warm and nourish the body. Try these offerings, and create your own.

High Prevention Dinner: The vegetable dish, and the broccoli in the noodle cakes, help boost your immunity to disease. In addition, the fruit in the pear sauce contains a compound called "pectin" that helps the digestive system eliminate toxins.

* Thyme-Roasted Vegetables (page 270)
* Chinese-Style Noodle Cakes (page 244)
* Warm Pear Sauce (page 299)

Decongesting Lunch or Dinner: If you've come down with a cold, the garlic and hot peppers in this meal will help open your stuffed head.

* Hot Pepper Salsa (with baked corn chips) (page 288)
* Spicy Bean Burritos (page 289)
* Breathe-Better Teas (pages 236–238)

Body-Boosting Breakfast: This high-fiber, low-fat morning meal will help keep you energized until lunch.

* Chewy Apple-Oat Bars (page 298)
* Cinnamon-Poached Fruit (page 294)

Tummy-Taming Dinner: If you have caught a seasonal stomach flu, this meal will help soothe your discomfort. Start out with half a serving of the millet dish, and eat slowly.

* Squash with Millet (page 284)
* Rosemary and Lavender Tisane (page 234)

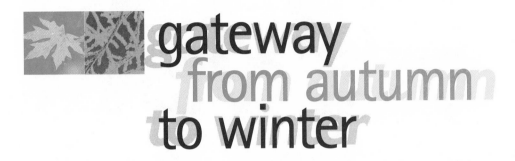

gateway
from autumn to winter

n ow is the time to begin the passage into the darker, inwardly directed season of winter. No matter what your climate—be it four full seasons, tropical, or desert—the days are shorter, the nights are longer, and the pressures of pending holidays can add up to oversensitivity and haywire emotions. Depression, anxiety, and irritability can be avoided, however, by staying grounded. Think of the roots of plants, firmly connected in the winter ground, resting, yet very much alive despite the weather. By staying grounded—or rooted, if you will—you stay connected to your Self. For instance, as one yoga instructor advises, when you feel off balance, take a walk outside. Go to a park, or look at the sky, but find something in nature that's bigger than your irritation. This process grounds you by framing the situations in your day in a larger perspective.

Another way to stay grounded is to calm your breathing. At the very moment you start to feel anxious or irritable, observe your breathing and try to deepen it. Close your eyes and breathe slowly ten times, counting down once, on each exhalation, from ten until you get to one. In this short time you will have performed a mini-meditation that may help circumvent a bad mood. The following suggestions may also help.

Mellow Music—To help you move smoothly into the season of rest, pay attention to what you listen to. Stock up on peaceful, soothing music that will assist you in being in harmony with the season, providing an audible, subtle message of grounding. Go for tinkling chimes, bells, flutes, and chorals, rather than screechy or dissonant selections.

Adopt an "Importance Index"—If you find yourself being pulled in too many directions and stressed by too many demands, make an "Importance Index." On a piece of paper, from the top down, write 5,4,3,2,1. Then rank your tasks. "Five" is the most important—an emergency. "Three" denotes an average situation, and "1" denotes a task that is not important at the moment. Weigh each situation that comes your way on your "Importance Index." If it's not a "4" or "5," it can wait until you have more time.

Cache of Candles—Buddhist meditators say that gazing quietly at the flame of a candle, even for five minutes, is grounding and balancing to the stressed soul. Stock up on candles and light one when you feel overwhelmed by the season. The flame is warming and provides a serene environment. Experiment with plain tapers, as well as with candles scented with comforting cinnamon, pine, or vanilla.

epilogue

How odd it must seem to have an epilogue—an ending—to a book that, for many pages, has taught that life is best lived from a cyclic point of view. Every ending has a beginning, every winter has a spring. But I'm writing this to remind you that as you go off to explore the cycles of the seasons, you may find it worthwhile to experiment with two key points: flexibility and open-mindedness.

Be flexible, because rigidity can make you ill. Think of leaving the house on a luscious spring day, wearing a light jacket. The day is warmer than you expected and you discover the jacket is making you feel overheated. What do you do? Take it off, of course. Conversely, if you remain too attached to the idea of wearing the jacket and leave it on, you'll be uncomfortable all day, which will lead to stress and its various physical manifestations. Go beyond your wardrobe with this analogy and try to be flexible emotionally as you move through life. Things that you've planned on will change, and being flexible—letting go of notions that no longer work for you or the situation—will keep you comfortable and happy in every season.

Of course, to be flexible you need to have an open mind, and that's the second key point. Staying open to new ideas can keep you young for many years. Imagine a person who eats meat and potatoes every day all year long until someone suggests the new idea of eating lighter in summer, to help cool the body and keep it energized. A person with an open mind will consider this reasonable notion and give it a try. Just as with food, be open to all new ideas that come your way, and adopt the ones that can help keep you happy and healthy.

Staying flexible and being open-minded will keep you balanced as you maneuver through the seasons. For example, on a hot summer day you may relish a plunge in a cool pond. The refreshing dip balances by cooling you off. Similarly, if you're in a heated argument, you can take a break to cool off. While "chilling out," try to think in a flexible, open-minded manner and you will more easily find a solution, or a balance, to your argument.

By adopting these techniques, you may find yourself becoming more peaceful and more cheerful. One woman told me that she first noticed a change while she was stuck in a huge traffic jam, late for an appointment. Suddenly she realized she was genuinely amused and not at all annoyed by her situation. She had a flexible and open attitude, and it worked in her favor. She also knew that the traffic jam—like all other situations—was cyclic, and would eventually evolve—not end but change into the beginning of something else, which in her case was a clear roadway.

In this same cyclic way, this book does not end, because you are using the ideas in it to help yourself be flexible and open-minded, and to create infinite new beginnings. As you travel through many seasons to come, may this always be true for you.

recipe index

SPRING

Cleansing Spring Beverages

Cleansing Spring Foods

SUMMER

Cooling Summer Beverages

Cooling Summer Foods

AUTUMN

Strengthening Autumn Beverages

Strengthening Autumn Foods

Apples and Pears

Broccoli

Cabbage

Cauliflower

Greens

Hot Peppers

Garlic and Onions

Orange-Fleshed Squash

general index

GENERAL INDEX